The benefits of Keto and Intermittent diet for 50+

Eva Bartlett

Copyright © 2022 by Eva Bartlett

All rights reserved.

No portion of this book may be reproduced in any form without written permission from the publisher or author, except as permitted by U.S. copyright law.

Contents

1.	Introduction	1
2.	Tips	15
3.	The diet	27
4.	My personal recipes	53

Chapter One

Introduction

A disclaimer: This material is for educational and entertaining purposes only, and should not be used for any other reason. We've made every effort to ensure that the information shown here is both up to date and comprehensive. Not one warranty is made or implied. Legal, financial, medical, or other professional advice is not being provided by the author. This book's content has been sourced from a variety of sources. Prior to attempting any of the strategies described in this book, you should get expert advice.

By reading this document, the reader accepts that under no circumstances is the author liable for any damages, direct or indirect, that are incurred as a consequence of the use of the information contained within this document, including, but not limited to, mistakes, omissions, or inaccuracies.

Women over the age of 50 who are interested in adopting and maintaining a Keto diet should read this guide. Over the last several years, you have certainly heard a lot about the Keto diet. If you've ever wanted to lose weight while still having fun, this is the diet for you. All ages have witnessed its great advantages.

Packed with meals that are rich in protein and high in fat and doing away with carbs is the ultimate way that the Keto diet assists you to lose weight and keep a healthy physique. Instead of burning carbs, your body will be educated to burn fats, improving your metabolism in an effective method. It also converts your lipids into ketones in your liver, which gives your brain an extra burst of fuel.

Instead of focusing on the carbs that you would be giving up, the Keto diet concentrates its attention on all of the protein and fats that your body desires. In an ideal world, you would be able to cook and enjoy your favourite dishes even while you're away from home. One of the advantages of the Keto diet is that it is one of the least restrictive diets out there. If you have any queries concerning the Keto diet, this guide will answer them all for you. You'll be surprised at how much flexibility you have on this diet compared to other diets. It's almost as if you're not even trying to lose weight.

When it comes to keeping your energy levels high as you become older, it's crucial to pay attention to all of the methods you may do so successfully. When you're running on half the energy you're used to, some jobs become a lot more difficult. Women, especially those over 50, do exceptionally well on the Keto diet. To top it all off, you'll see a reduction in inflammation and an even distribution of your hormones, which will improve your overall well-being. Your physical and mental well-being will improve as a result of these advantages. Your mental health is also a major factor to keep in mind when dieting. Many diets make you feel deprived of the foods you crave, which can lead to a downbeat frame of mind.

This tutorial will explain why keto is so different from other diets. It's a way of living that practically anybody can adopt, no matter what their typical day looks like. You'll be brimming with the confidence and positivity you need to achieve your objectives. Keto can help you achieve your goals, whether they're to maintain your current weight or lose weight. It will become an anti-aging diet that will become a part of your daily routine.

As you embark on your personal Keto adventure, you'll reap the following fantastic rewards:

Long-term shedding of pounds

Reduced amounts of blood sugar

Increased stamina

Skin that seems more youthful.

By increasing the body's metabolic rate

Well-functioning hormone systems

From the inside out, anti-aging advantages.

A broad array of mouthwatering dishes to choose from.

INTRODUCTION 3

Keto is a diet that most women can adapt to quickly and easily, and they have no difficulty sticking to it. All of your Keto-related queries will be addressed in this comprehensive resource.

If you want to feel and look your best, then the Keto diet is for you. It'll be a diet unlike any other since you'll feel terrific during the entire process. To be successful on the diet, you don't need to use any gimmicks or deceptive methods. The Keto diet may be easily integrated into your present lifestyle if you are knowledgeable about what to consume. So, let's get started and find out what the Keto diet is all about and how it may benefit you!

How did the ketogenic diet come to be?

In order to maintain a state of "fasting" in your body, the Keto diet focuses on eliminating simple carbohydrates and increasing fat intake. Ketosis is a state in which your body begins to burn ketones, rather than glucose, rather than glucose. According to the majority of experts, this will improve your health without having to restrict the amount of food that you consume on an everyday basis.

For the most part, the diet adheres to a 60-75 percent healthy fat intake, 1530 percent protein consumption, and barely 5-10 percent carbohydrate consumption plan. Because it appears to be a diet with little restrictions, many people are hesitant at first. However, the diet is really that easy.

The ultimate objective of the keto diet is to put your body into a state of ketosis. Glucose, a kind of sugar, is the primary source of energy for your body. When carbohydrates are removed from your diet, your body experiences "starvation," but this is a false sense of hunger. As a result, your body will begin to make the required modifications to refocus its energy. To maintain the glucose flowing to the brain, it will then produce a supplementary energy source generated from fat. As a result of the lack of carbohydrates, your body will use the fat components as a fuel source instead of glucose.

This diet has proven to be quite effective for a large number of people. You'll not only lose weight, but you'll also feel better and have more energy than you've had in a long time. The term "ketogenic" is a relatively recent invention, having first appeared in the early twentieth century. The Ancient Greeks, on the other hand, advocated tight diets as a treatment for epilepsy long before this name was used. It's a fascinating history that merits a cursory look.

4   THE BENEFITS OF KETO AND INTERMITTENT DIET FOR 50+

Fasting was the sole known cure for epilepsy in Hippocrates' day. After two thousand years, this became an almost universal habit. It spread from Europe to the rest of the world at a rapid pace. Today, most individuals follow the Ketogenic diet to lose weight and improve their health, however the diet's beginnings plainly declare that it was intended to change the way the brain works. When compared to people on a conventional diet, epileptic patients on the Keto diet in 1911 had fewer seizures and less symptoms. A few weeks of consistent fasting yielded these outcomes.

Dr. Hugh Conklin, an osteopathic physician in the United States, began recommending fasting as a therapy approach for his epileptic patients about the same period. At one point, they were fasting for 18-25 days in a row, and the results were astounding. Adult patients reported a 50% success rate, whereas paediatric patients reported a 90% success rate. Of course, this is an extreme form of the processed diet that we are familiar with today. Although the outcomes were outstanding, health practitioners were aware that this was not a long-term solution. Temporary fasting is inherent in the practise. Seizures would reoccur as soon as the patients resumed their usual meals.

Doctors began working on a long-term therapy strategy as soon as they realised this issue existed. As a result, doctors began to focus on removing certain sugars and carbohydrates in order to better understand these consequences. In the research, Dr. Wilder, a well-known Mayo Clinic physician, was a participant. His patients were experiencing less seizures as their blood sugar levels dropped. Dr. Wilder is credited with establishing the Ketogenic diet as a permanent lifestyle rather than a short-term therapy method. Everyday eating patterns now match the way your metabolism works when you're fasting.

From a simple idea, we've developed a straightforward diet strategy. For the most part, patients didn't notice they were starving themselves throughout their prolonged fasts. When you alter your diet to include more ketones, your body responds instantly. In this way, people may fool their bodies into thinking they were starving while still obtaining all of the calories and nourishment they required. Ketosis was given a major boost because to this amazing finding.

In addition to Dr. M.G. Peterman, another Mayo Clinic specialist, the diet was standardised by him. A "classic keto" strategy, he said. This strategy is still widely employed today. Maintaining a 4:1 fat to protein and carbohydrate ratio is essential. 90 percent of all calories come from fat, while 6 percent come from protein and only 4 percent from carbohydrates. This is frequently regarded of as an optimum approach to the Keto diet, but a 3:1 ratio is also considered extremely advantageous. This might sound excessive on paper, but it genuinely isn't hard to sustain since your body still knows that it is getting all of the nourishment that it requires.

There is often one significant concern that remains after reading about the Keto diet, and that surrounds what you can really consume. While on a diet, the following foods were considered essential:

Onions, garlic, and peppers are examples of vegetables that do not contain starch.

Full Fat Dairy Products: Cheese, yoghurt, and milk

Eggs, soybeans, shellfish, fish, pork, chicken, and cattle are all sources of protein.

Almonds, pistachios, walnuts, sunflower seeds, and pumpkin seeds are some of the most popular nuts and seeds.

All sources of high-quality fats are available, from plants and animals alike.

A few of my favourite fruits include avocado, rhubarb, coconut, and blueberries. "

In order to get the best outcomes, doctors would stress the need of utilising exact measurements. These ratios were to be closely monitored. The meal had to be measured to the gramme before each patient could eat it since it had become so exact. That mimicking fasting diet could be maintained for extended periods of time was evident to doctors.

Even now, more than two centuries later, the Keto diet is mostly intact. Participants should ingest one gramme of protein for every kilogramme of their body weight, according to nutritionists. Carbohydrate consumption should be limited to 10-15 grammes per day, with the balance of the diet concentrated on consuming fats.

It's still a mystery why the Keto diet has been so effective for epileptics, scientifically speaking. Ketones are thought to produce an anti-electrical reaction in the brain because of their inherent composition. Because they are no longer exposed to these electrical currents, those who suffer from seizures are no longer at risk of having them again. It's exciting to consider the outcomes for epileptic patients, but the advantages go well beyond that. Doctors quickly realised that the Keto diet may help people who weren't epileptics as well.

Incredibly, this revelation was made during a study of the food on youngsters. Kids on the diet were shown to be less abrasive and more focused than those who were not. They were also expected to sleep better at night, which would have been an additional advantage. In the 2000s, more study was carried out, and it came to the same conclusion. Anticonvulsant medications have made the feeding technique obsolete. Only lately has the Keto diet been recognised as a viable diet and lifestyle choice.

When the Keto diet was put on hold, it lost a lot of its lustre. As a result, many people misapplied it, failing to adhere to its exact specifications. Fewer dieticians had prior expertise with the regimen, therefore they were ill-equipped to help their patients stick to it correctly. People's perceptions of the Keto diet were tainted by their poor experiences with it. In only a few decades, the Keto diet acquired a negative connotation connected to it that made it unappealing to many individuals. During this time, the Keto diet began to fade away as a therapy or diet option.

Reassessing the Ketogenic Diet

In the 1990s, the ketogenic diet was once again popular. Many people remained fascinated by it, not because it was a diet to follow, but because of the mystifying nature of its operation. A few of these episodes aired before a 1994 broadcast of Dateline, a news show, brought some good attention to the Keto diet.

A two-year-old toddler was the focus of the show. He had suffered from severe epilepsy for a long time. Before starting the Keto diet, his seizures were out of control. While it was a dangerous manoeuvre, it was the only option John Hopkins doctors had. They went to Keto because of the seriousness of his condition. Fewer than ten children were being treated for epilepsy in this manner annually at the time.

People in the medical community and the general public alike were outraged when the episode aired. Scientific curiosity has skyrocketed as well. A renewed interest in the Keto diet set everything in motion once more. A video called "First Do No Harm" was even made by the child's father as a result of this. The movie, which starred Meryl Streep and was released in 1997, is about a couple's experience with a special diet and the positive impact it had on their kid. The fact that it was shown on national television only served to amplify interest in the subject.

INTRODUCTION   7

There has been a resurgence of interest in Keto, which has brought us to the modern-day experience of the diet. Once again, hospitals offered it as a viable therapy option. When the Keto diet was initially introduced, epilepsy was treated in the same way. Almost all major children's hospitals employ the Keto diet as a treatment regimen nowadays. Because of its significance in treating neurological problems, it continues to draw scientific and medical attention. There's more to the tale, though.

If the Keto diet was exclusively helpful for those with epilepsy, it's possible that interest in it would have waned by now. A lot of individuals have come to recognise how great the diet is for regulating physical health and weight management since its return to the spotlight. Those seeking a more healthy way of life began to take notice of the Keto diet with this shift in attitude. Because of this resurgence of interest in Keto, scientists discovered that it may be utilised purely as a dietary strategy for those with perfect neurological health.

Keto took some time to gain traction as a diet that can be relied upon by those without epilepsy. The Atkins diet was also making a comeback in the 1990s. If you've been paying attention to dietary fads over the last several decades, you've probably heard of the Atkins diet. This diet plan has a similar perspective on carbohydrates, and the way it was presented really took off during this period of time. Despite the fact that Atkins was the diet of choice for the general public, this gave scientists and researchers greater leeway to investigate Keto on its own as a viable alternative. Making place for the diet that we now know so much more about, the two were often compared to one other.

Keto has progressively displaced Atkins as the fashionable diet du jour. As a result, many individuals considered Atkins to be extremely restrictive and difficult. It was difficult for individuals on the diet to eat out or away from home. Keto intended to alter people's perceptions of food. Those who tried it realised that they could reduce weight while maintaining a healthy lifestyle. Being on Keto doesn't seem like a diet at all, according to many. Instead, it serves as a manual for how we should care for our bodies, outlining a straightforward approach. Because you don't have to calculate calories every single day, Keto is a lot of fun. A more adaptable eating plan, it helps people to maintain their sense of self-identity.

Furthermore, Keto is flourishing in an age when social media is so widely used. It has proven itself to dietitians and the general public alike. It's simple for Keto dieters to keep tabs on their progress in real time, which is both reassuring and enlightening. It's unusual to see posts regarding the Keto diet on any of the major social media networks. Additionally, many individuals prefer to post photos of their cuisine online! While the internet expanded our access to information in the early 2000s, the present decade allows us to go even deeper into our knowledge. It's easier to relate to Keto after reading about other people's real-life experiences with it. It also provides us with ideas for foods and ways to enjoy the ketogenic diet.

Observe how your body feels. That's the simple message. If you don't know exactly how to implement and apply a new diet plan to your personal life, it can be a bit of a gamble. The research behind the Keto diet continues to astonish people from all walks of life and all corners of the globe. As soon as you begin your Keto diet, you'll notice a noticeable change in your physique. This is because of what's going on inside the organisation. Keto does not promise speedy or unrealistic weight loss, unlike many other gimmick diets or fads. Instead, it provides an overall lifestyle solution that can be followed by anyone.

Regardless of whether or not you are ready to begin your own Keto adventure, the outcomes will speak for themselves. As we become older, our bodies naturally begin to decline. As a result, we may get caught up in the newest health fads and wind up eating things we don't particularly like. In the beginning, it's crucial to be open-minded about Keto. As long as you pay attention to your body, eat in quantities that are familiar to you, and experiment with your meals, you'll discover that the Keto diet is a positive addition to your life and diet.

Women in their 50s are more mindful of their general health than they were when they were younger. And it's quite normal to feel that way. This book's goal is to assist you in putting your newfound knowledge into action, especially through utilising the advantages of a Ketogenic diet. While making a change in your life may seem simple, there are a few things you should know before taking the plunge, which we'll go over in detail in this book. Ketogenic diets come in a wide variety of forms and methods. As a result, we'll begin there.

SKD, TKD, and CKD are all types of Ketogenic diets.

The ability to stick to a diet plan is much enhanced when you have some degree of diet flexibility. By looking into the numerous varieties of the Keto diet, you may learn more about the origins of the diet and how it differs from other types. If you don't want to follow a predetermined path, realise that there are alternatives.

INTRODUCTION 9

In reality, there are three methods to tailor the ketogenic diet to your own needs. Now you can eat whatever you want without feeling like you're restricting yourself in any way. With these alternatives, most other diet regimens appear more restrictive. Everybody's needs are different, and Keto wants to help everyone find a diet that works best for them.

The main difference between these two types of Keto is in the percentages of the items you'll be consuming. While they all agree on the fundamental principle of cutting off carbohydrates in order to achieve ketosis, there are several strategies to do this. A breadless diet, for example, doesn't mean you'll always be grouchy because you may consume carbohydrates at particular times of the day in some variations of the diet. Try each of the three options and discover which one works best for your body type. It's possible that your decision will be influenced by what you've been consuming before. It is fantastic since moving between these three types is neither severe or harmful. They differ just enough to provide you alternatives without jeopardising your health in the process.

Strictly Keto Diet (SKD):

If you've heard of the Keto diet, you've probably heard of the conventional Keto diet. It is the most popular plan since it gives a solid foundation and introduction to the lifestyle. Low-carbohydrate, moderate-protein diet is the focus of this diet plan. All efforts are aimed towards maintaining a high-fat diet.

In this case, the individual consumes 75% fat, 20% protein, and 5% carbohydrates. (This will serve as your daily general guideline.) Because these simple concepts are so easy to remember once you become used to them, this strategy is popular with many people. Research on the SKD has been the most comprehensive. Researchers are most likely referring to the SKD approach when they talk about Keto.

Effective weight loss is only one of the many advantages this supplement has to offer. When embarking on a new diet, this is a major issue for many people. You may lose weight securely and healthily with the SKD if you so want. For this diet to function, there are no strong hunger pangs as you would on other diets. When on the Keto diet, you should never feel like you are genuinely starving yourself. The body's desire to deviate from the plan is the outcome of this bad sensation. At some point in your diet journey, you've undoubtedly experienced this firsthand. It's easy to succumb to the temptation to consume unhealthy meals that "comfort" you if you're hungry enough. Losing momentum in this manner may be demoralising.

Another advantage of being on the SKD is that your chances of contracting illnesses and disorders are reduced. Keto's goal is to guide you toward a healthier lifestyle by providing a well-balanced diet. While on the diet, you won't be preoccupied with calorie monitoring or food restriction, so you'll be able to enjoy this perk to its fullest. Because it differs so greatly from a low-fat diet, the ketogenic way of eating is so satisfying. You'll be less prone to wander since your body is getting enough protein. According to one study, the Keto diet has a weight reduction success rate up to 2.2 times greater than other comparable diets.

When beginning the Keto diet, keep your diabetes risk factors in mind. There's a chance that this risk factor will go up with age. Changing your metabolism and spiking your blood sugar are two of the most common issues. Your metabolism is redirected, and your blood sugar levels are maintained, according to the SKD, as you are aware. As a result of your body burning harmful fats that aren't required for its proper functioning while on the Keto diet, you will lose weight. As a result, you'll lose weight and get rid of extra fat you don't need. Those who are pre-diabetic or have a family history of diabetes might considerably benefit from the ketogenic diet.

In addition, there are other more advantages. Cancer, heart disease, Alzheimer's disease, and polycystic ovarian syndrome are just a few of the diseases that the SKD has been shown to help prevent. Many, if not all, of these illnesses have elevated risks associated with advancing age. Considering that Keto has the potential to protect you from all of these ailments is astounding. You'll feel wonderful about your trip if you don't give up all of your favourite meals. As you plan your meals and consider what other elements of your life need to adapt to accommodate your new eating habits, remembering that Keto is not only beneficial but also preventive may help you stay motivated. While on Keto, it's not difficult to remember what to do. You're enabling your body to acclimate to the diet naturally if you avoid sugary foods, natural or manufactured. You won't even realise that you're cutting off carbs if you focus on making meat and dairy taste great. Targeted Ketogenic Diet (TKD)

The Keto diet is tailored to your specific fitness routines. In addition to adhering to a healthy eating plan, you should also make a concerted effort to exercise and get your body moving. While the SKD does not require carbohydrates prior to workouts, the TKD does require carbs. As a result, your physical health might take precedence over your mental well-being. In order to stay healthy as you become older, it's important to increase the quantity of activity you engage in. Even if you may not be able to do the activities you used to when you were younger, this does not negate the importance of maintaining a healthy weight and physical fitness. In the forefront, participating in TKD necessitates a rigorous physical regimen.

Before you start changing your eating habits, you'll need to do some pre-work to make this strategy work for you. Take a moment to think about the workouts you love and that are appropriate for your current level of fitness. In order to avoid going overboard, it's important to start small and work your way up from there. Building a healthy diet around regular exercise might begin with light to moderate activity two or three times per week. On the days you plan to workout, eat carbohydrates and stick to the Keto diet for the other five days of the week. This programme is designed for people who are committed to a regular exercise regimen. If you eat according to the TKD approach without exercising, it will show you negative impacts.

Even if you're on the TKD diet, you can still have a weight loss objective in mind. The most important thing to keep in mind is to not overindulge yourself while you're on carb-loading days. Because you'll be restricting the amount of carbs you give your body, keep in mind that they'll be counted as calories. Because of this, you'll need to modify your fat intake on those days as well. The most difficult element of learning the TKD is figuring out how to keep everything in balance. As far as exercise and carb intake go, you're the only one who can keep yourself accountable. A little trial and error is usual when it comes to getting this ratio just perfect.

In between the SKD and CKD, the TKD serves as a bridge. As long as you don't overdo it, you can stay in ketosis for a long time. Training in TKD has been demonstrated to increase stamina and help you to make real progress toward your fitness objectives for many people. If you're just getting started with the Keto diet, this is a good option for you. Incorporating this strategy into your daily routine might have several advantages if you're open to the idea. As a result, you are able to set more ambitious exercise objectives, demonstrating another another benefit of the Keto diet: it is not restrictive.

Exercising will get less taxing as time passes. This is an excellent time to examine your fitness plan and determine if it's still appropriate for your current situation. However, you should avoid making frequent dietary changes and instead focus on gradually increasing the intensity of your TKD workouts. Be aware that this is only an option it presents. There's no need to make any adjustments if your body is functioning normally and your endurance is increasing. For the first month or so of your diet plan, you should not make any significant dietary changes. Consuming carbohydrates 30 minutes before exercise is ideal. When it comes to fueling their exercises, many people find that between 25 and 50 grammes of carbohydrates is ideal. CKD: Cyclical Ketogenic Dieting

The CKD approach, as previously said, is the type of Keto that is most likely to have fluctuations in results. You will alternate between a low-carbohydrate, high-fat diet and a high-carbohydrate diet on this diet plan. This version of Keto is the most regimented of all the others. You will let your body "refeeding days" when you have CKD. In order to refill your body's glucose levels, you will eat more carbohydrates on certain days of the week. When it comes to building muscle, the CKD is a popular choice. Bodybuilders and others who take their workouts seriously often use this strategy. Be aware, however, that the CKD has the least amount of research backing it of all the forms of Keto that are now followed.

Carb cycling and chronic kidney disease (CKD) are often confused, although they are not the same thing. Carb cycling involves decreasing carbohydrates for a period of time and then refilling your body's carbohydrate stores for the remainder of the week. A typical week is divided into 4-6 days of low-carb eating and 1-3 days of high-carbohydrate consumption. You can't go into ketosis on a carb cycling diet, whereas the CKD does. Because of this, you won't be able to get the full benefits of the Keto diet.

Even though this is the type of Keto diet that you are least likely to benefit from, it is still worth learning about because it is one that a large number of people adhere to. Basically, the person must eat no more than 50 grammes of carbohydrates a day on average. About 75% of your diet should consist of lipids that are good for you. Avocados, eggs, dairy products, nut butters, and fatty meats are some of the alternatives. This diet has a protein content of roughly 15%. Carbohydrates can be consumed in greater quantities on refeeding days. About 60% of your total calories will come from carbohydrates, with protein and fat accounting for the remaining 20% and 5%, respectively. As you can see, there is a considerable difference between normal and re-feeding days.

On refeeding days, it's a widespread misperception that people on the CKD consume a lot of bread to receive their carbohydrates. However, this is neither the norm or a healthy suggestion. Sweet potatoes, butternut squash, brown rice, quinoa, oats, and other whole-grain foods are commonly used in the CKD approach. On those days, as you can see, discipline is still essential, despite the increased carb consumption. There is a lot of vitamin and nutritional content

INTRODUCTION 13

in all of these carbohydrates. Sugary and artificial foods and beverages are still discouraged since they do not provide any nutritional value. The CKD is probably not the diet for you if you don't intend to match it with a somewhat tough exercise programme and routine.

We also recommend including some intermittent fasting into your CKD regimen. Following the days of refeeding, you will fast for short periods of time. This will speed up your return to ketosis. To get the most out of ketosis and maximise muscle gain, your exercises should be done after your refeeding days. If you're only want to lose weight or slow the effects of ageing, the CKD isn't for you. It's just a more intense form of Keto. To be sure, CKD can be beneficial to those who consistently engage in high-intensity training on a weekly basis or who want to do so in the near future.

When it comes to sports or other physical activities, the biggest advantage of the CKD technique is the possibility for muscle growth and endurance strengthening. The varying refeeding days might lead to constipation in those on the CKD, which is a drawback. It is essential to monitor your fibre intake and ensure that you are well hydrated in order to prevent this. You should aim to keep up with the SKD diet for a few months before transitioning to the CKD, which is a major commitment in terms of dieting.

SKD, TKD, or CKD are all viable options, depending on your present health and your long-term health objectives. As a general rule, the Ketogenic diet may be used by persons with a wide range of aims and objectives. Why, therefore, is the Keto diet ideal for women over the age of fifty? Next, we'll look into it.

Why Women in their 50s?

Chapter Two

Tips

If you're a woman, you've probably noticed that dieting for women differs significantly from dieting for males. Because of the way their hormones work and the way their bodies burn down fat, women often have a more difficult time losing weight than men do. Consider your age group as well. As we grow older, it becomes increasingly necessary to take better care of our bodies. Diet and exercise can delay the onset of many of the issues that accompany ageing. Keto is effective for women of all ages because of the way it interacts with the body's natural systems. Keto will alter your body's metabolism in a way that is unique to you, no matter how fit you are or how much weight you need to lose.

You shouldn't think about going to extremes while starting a Keto diet since that's not what Keto is supposed to be about. To put your body into ketosis, you should be able to do it without feeling bad. When you first begin your Keto journey, one of the most important rules to remember is to pay close attention to your body's signals. If you ever feel hungry or unsatisfied, you may need to change your diet since you aren't achieving ketosis effectively. Be patient with yourself and your body since this is a long-term process. It takes some time and awareness to adjust to a Keto diet. Because it's a safe diet for women to follow.

The health advantages of the Keto diet are not different for men or women, but the speed at which they are attained does change. As noted, women's bodies are a lot different when it comes to the methods that they are able to burn fats and lose weight. For example, by design women have at least 10 percent more body fat than males. No matter how fit you are, this is just a facet of being a woman that you must consider. Don't be harsh on yourself if you realise that it looks like males can lose weight easily - that's because they can! Men, on the other hand, tend to have more muscular mass than women. Because they have more muscular mass, males tend to notice better effects on the outside because their metabolisms are faster. That higher metabolism implies that fat and energy is expended quicker. When you are on Keto, though, the internal transformation is happening immediately away.

You have a distinct metabolism, but it is also slower than a man's. Because muscle burns more calories than fat, males are able to attain their potential for muscular growth far more quickly than women. In no way, shape, or form, should this deter you from embarking on your Keto adventure. You won't be baffled as to why it's taking you so long to start losing weight if you keep these physiological realities in mind. You will eventually reach this position, but it will take some time and effort on your part to get there.

Polycystic Ovary Syndrome (PCOS), or Polycystic Ovary Syndrome, is a hormonal imbalance that causes cysts to form in the ovaries of women. It is possible that these cysts will rupture, causing serious harm to the female reproductive system. As many as 10% of the female population is affected with PCOS, making it one of the most frequent female conditions. Quite a few ladies are unaware that they have the disorder. PCOS is undetected in over 70% of women. This illness can lead to a substantial hormonal imbalance, which might have an impact on your metabolism and energy expenditure. As a result, dieting becomes even more difficult because weight gain is inevitable. Regular visits to the gynaecologist are essential for maintaining good health.

We all have to deal with menopause at some point in our lives, especially as we become older. Menopause typically begins in the mid-40s for the majority of women. The slowing of the metabolism and weight gain associated with menopause do not affect males since they do not go through menopause. Menopause is a time when it's easy to gain weight and lose muscle. Most women, once menopause begins, lose muscle at a much faster rate, and conversely gain weight, despite dieting and exercise regimens. Because of this, the ketogenic diet may be the best option for you. What ever your body does naturally, such as menopause, your internal systems will still move from running on carbohydrates to getting their energy from fat.

Having the ability to run on fats means you have an automated fuel reserve that may be used at any time. When your body learns to use the fat you currently have for energy, you will be able to consume less calories while still feeling satisfied. This will take some time to happen. This will soon become second nature to you. In the end, patience is required, but being aware of what your body is telling you can keep you going while on Keto.

Diabetes-related insulin resistance can be prevented since the Keto diet limits sugar intake. For women with PCOS and reproductive concerns, as well as menopause symptoms and illnesses like pre-diabetes and Type 2 diabetes, this can have a positive impact. Once your body becomes used to the keto diet, you'll be able to overcome the natural barriers to weight loss and good health that may be standing in your way. A tight diet may not have the same benefits as embarking on the Keto diet since your body isn't getting rid of sugars correctly. For women, it's a significant reason why Keto is so good.

In the past, we've talked about the importance of carbohydrates and sugar in affecting your hormonal balance. In order to discover that your hormones are out of whack, you may need an entirely new way of eating. When you embark on a ketogenic diet, your hormones will be restored to a healthy range. A brighter outlook on life and greater energy to get through the day are likely outcomes of this.

It is recommended that women over the age of 50 start their Keto diet under the guidance of a physician. In the long run, if you stick to the plan and pay attention to your body's demands, you won't have any more troubles than males have. There will be more challenges ahead of you, but you can conquer them. Keep in mind that a large number of women have had wonderful success on a low-carb, high-fat diet. Use the stories of these ladies as a guide for your own path. Keep in mind the things that are working against you, but also the things that are working in your favour. Rather than storing fat as a result of ingesting carbohydrates, your body is more suited to entering ketosis. Use this as a nudge to keep going, and you'll get there. For those over 50, keto is a viable alternative, and the outcomes will show it.

Is it safe for those over 50 to go on a low-carb diet?

It's only natural that as we become older, we'd like to hang on to our youthful vitality and vitality. If you're thinking about anti-aging, you're not alone. Everywhere you look, there are ads for products and lifestyle modifications aimed at grabbing your attention as you face the realities of being a woman over 50 in today's culture. It is probable that you have thought about anti-aging nutrition in other ways, such as the way you care for your skin and hair. The Keto diet is fantastic because it promotes optimal health from the inside out, working tirelessly to ensure that you are in the finest form possible.

Indigestion is an example of a typical ailment that occurs as you become older. This occurs as a result of the body's decreased ability to break down specific nutrients. We've all gotten used to putting up with our bodies going through agony in order to digest normal meals because of all the chemicals and fillers. The Keto diet will make you conscious of how your digestion has begun to alter, even if you aren't aware of what you're doing to your body. Afterwards, you will no longer feel bloated or ill at ease. It's probable that you're overeating and gaining weight because you're not getting the nutrition you need from the food you're consuming.

Your body is able to fully absorb and assimilate all of the nutrients that you consume through the keto diet. You should not feel the urge to overeat in order to compensate for a lack of nutrients when you consume your meals. Anti-aging is anything that reduces the stress on any part of your body. Once you begin your Keto journey, you will rapidly notice this advantage, since it is one of the first improvements that most participants mention. Additionally, you'll be able to go to the toilet more frequently, without experiencing any of the issues that are typically linked with ageing.

Most 50+ women who begin a diet plan want to lose weight, but the method by which they do it matters. If you've ever lost a significant amount of weight, you've likely encountered the unpleasant side effects of sagging or drooping skin. The skin's elasticity improves by following a ketogenic diet. Your skin will be able to keep up with you as you lose weight. Keto dieters don't have to put in a lot of effort to tighten up their skin, since it should already be doing so each day. It's a nice surprise for many individuals to learn this information.

Another typical benefit reported by women is a decrease in wrinkles and an improvement in their overall health, including hair and skin development. It is common for women who begin the diet to remark that their ageing process really slows down. In addition to looking and feeling better, the skin also gets firmer. The effects of Keto on your skin and face can be appreciated even if you aren't currently reducing weight.. To indicate that you're getting healthier from the inside out, you'll look better in no time. Because of this, you'll begin to feel better, as well. You may read about others' experiences, but nothing compares to experiencing it for yourself when you embark on a Keto diet.

We all have daily duties that tyre us and require a certain level of energy to do, especially ladies over the age of 50. Even if you get adequate sleep at night, ageing can deplete your energy reserves, which is a sad fact. It imposes restrictions on how you may live your life, which can be demoralising. As an example, most diets lead to fatigue, which participants are instructed to become accustomed to. Keto, on the other hand, has the exact opposite effect. Increasing your energy levels is one of the many benefits of following the Keto diet instructions. Since your body is receiving all of the nutrients it requires, it will reward you with an abundance of energy.

The increased sensitivity of one's blood sugar levels, which many women over 50 experience almost overnight, is another prevalent concern. Those over the age of 50 should pay particular attention to their blood pressure and cholesterol readings, but everyone should be aware of them. High blood sugar can be a warning sign of diabetes, but as we've already established, adopting a Keto diet can serve as a preventative measure. In addition, managing increased blood sugar levels naturally lowers systemic inflammation, which is especially frequent in women over the age of 50. – Common aches and pains can be eased by restoring harmony to the immune system, of which inflammation is a part. A common cause of joint stiffness is a natural inflammation of the joints, even if you've been working out and stretching regularly. Inflammation can also impair key organs and is a precursor to cancer. Keto will help you on your way to a healthier living.

Sugar is never good for us, but as we get older, it becomes even more harmful. A "sugar sag" can develop as you age due to an accumulation of sugar molecules on your skin and protein in your body. Even if you don't eat a lot of sugar, this can happen. The weakening of your proteins, which are intended to hold you together, might also be a cause of this drooping when you consume an average amount of sugar. More wrinkles and arterial stiffness accompany sagging.

The Keto diet may be able to alleviate any anti-aging problems you have. It's a diet that pushes you to your physical and mental limits while giving you a clear and concise set of rules to follow. There will be no "wrongs" or "breaks" in your relationship with Keto as long as you remain committed to your goals and remain motivated throughout the process. There are many ways you may lose weight on the diet if you know how to give up sugary foods and beverages while still ingesting the right quantity of carbohydrates.

The easy procedures that optimise your body to absorb extra fats for energy can help you feel better, look better, and have more energy as a woman over 50. You'll get stronger, slimmer, and younger as a result of your workouts. Many of the signs and symptoms associated with menopause can be alleviated or reversed by following a Ketogenic diet, as we've already discussed. In the following chapter, we'll see how.

Invigorate and Rejuvenate Your Body

Earlier in this chapter, you learned a little bit about how the ketogenic diet can improve your hormones and energy levels. Due to your daily dependence on these two items, this diet is going to make you feel fantastic. Nothing is more discouraging than embarking on a diet only to discover that it saps your energy and motivation. Doing keto correctly will not leave you feeling depressed. When you notice an increase in your energy, you've done everything you need to. As a result, your hormones will begin to return to their normal range. In your daily life, you may experience an increase in contentment and well-being as a result of this.

Women going through menopause, in particular, are familiar with the aggravating effects of hormonal imbalance. You've probably experienced it all in a short period of time, from hot flashes to mood swings. Discouragement can set in because it appears as if nothing is working. As a last resort, many women who are currently going through this are trying Keto as a desperate attempt to level the playing field. If your symptoms are severe, Keto has been shown to alleviate them and make life more bearable for those who have tried it.

In part, this is due to a rise in fat consumption: Because your body is literally changing the way it stores and breaks down fat, Keto allows you to consume more fat than you have ever been encouraged to do before. A higher intake of these healthy fats will prompt your body to produce more oestrogen and progesterone. To put it another way, reducing your fat intake may actually worsen hormonal imbalances already present in your body without you even being aware of it.

Keto's detoxification benefits women who are still experiencing menstrual cramps. When the body reaches this point of detoxification, PMS symptoms are reduced. An excess of oestrogen occurs during PMS, which makes it difficult to cope with the symptoms. For years, you've been dealing with cramping, bloating, and mood swings when you have too much oestrogen in your body. In some cases, this oestrogen dominance can be more pronounced when your diet is high in sugar. Additional progesterone is required to restore your hormonal equilibrium. Because the Keto diet cleanses and purifies your body, it will begin to replace the excess hormones that you don't need with the ones that you do.

As previously discussed, many women are unaware that they have PCOS. However, even if fertility isn't an issue for you any longer, living with PCOS has a slew of unwelcome consequences as you age. Unfortunately, there is no treatment for this disorder, so keeping it under control is absolutely essential.

With PCOS, poor blood sugar control and excess body fat can make this condition even worse. As a way to alleviate some of the symptoms of PCOS, many people have turned to the ketogenic diet. Everyone who followed the diet in a Duke University study was able to lose weight, and those who were hoping to improve their fertility were able to do so as well.

Insulin is a massive hormone that plays a critical role in your body's functioning. This regulates your blood sugar, which can affect your sex hormone levels if your blood sugar drops too far. As a result of going on the Keto diet, your body becomes more sensitive to insulin. Your cells will be able to appropriately utilise insulin if you have a healthy level of the hormone in your body. Studies have shown that up to 75% of obese diabetics have shown an improvement in insulin sensitivity as a result. These results are encouraging in that they yield a sizable number. Having a higher insulin sensitivity makes it easier for you to become in shape. You'll be able to keep the weight off more easily if you lose weight. Your risk of cardiovascular disease and dementia is reduced as a result of this,

With no break from stress, it is easy to feel exhausted in a short period of time. To keep up with the pressures in your life, your adrenal glands will release cortisol, which helps you feel more alert. When things get tough, your body tries to give you a little additional oomph to get you through it. However, your body may begin to create excessive amounts of cortisol as a result of this. You'll also be missing out on vital oestrogen and progesterone.

Cortisol is really harmful to your sex life, your muscle mass, and your general level of exhaustion, despite what your body believes it is doing to alleviate stress. In this situation, the body is more vulnerable, and Keto tries to supply you with a more moderate approach. If you don't want to feel like you can't get through the day, don't allow your body overcompensate for what it believes it needs. The Keto diet will help you get back on track and lead you down the correct path.

Diets low in fat provide poorer outcomes, as you will soon discover. Keto differs from most other diets in that it places a strong emphasis on not include these fats in the diet. Cutting out fats may sound like a reasonable request, but when your body is left with only carbs and sugars to absorb, this is really going to be damaging to your weight reduction, your general health, and your hormones will be thrown out of wack. Many people reach this conclusion only after exhausting a seemingly endless number of diet options. In the end, the Keto diet is meant to be a long-term solution for your weight-loss goals.

Overwhelmed with exhaustion

In the event that you frequently find yourself exhausted, the Keto diet may be a good option for you. Stressors and duties that people face each day might vary widely, yet the body's response to them can be vastly different. So it stands to reason that what you put into your body is quite vital for making it through each day; after all, food is fuel. Most of us end the day exhausted, but this doesn't have to be your default state of mind. Your body will really produce more energy than ever before if you feed it the appropriate nourishment.

It's possible to get long-lasting energy from keto, rather than just short spurts. Getting your energy from coffee or sugar, for example, just gives you a short burst of energy before you fall. This is because the energy is only supposed to last for a short period of time, and while it can get you through a short period of time, it isn't going to keep you going for the entire day. It is the more long-lasting energy that Keto provides. It's the type of energy that steadily builds up and never leaves you feeling depleted.

As a result of the SAD, carbohydrates are overconsumed. Most Americans overindulge in simple carbohydrates and fats that are bad for their health. While protein and carbohydrates make up most of a meal, healthy fats are almost always absent. Even more so, we are junk food addicts, eating far too many pre-packaged foods that are often loaded with carbohydrates and unhealthy fats, as well as eating sugary "health" foods like yoghurt and eating out at restaurants that serve huge portions of food that are laden with carbohydrates and fat, as well as sugar. These starches will be transformed to glucose or sugar molecules as a result of the excessive consumption of the improper sort of carbohydrates.

Based on your understanding of how the body operates while it is not on a Keto diet, you may infer that your body will simply absorb the glucose and use it as energy. This is when the issue of dwindling energy supplies really becomes apparent. Insulin is required to bring this process to a successful conclusion. Glucose levels increase, and so does insulin. This additional energy (glucose) is stored in your body even after you've consumed plenty. Additionally, insulin serves as a signal to your liver, letting it know that the glucose reserves in your body have been depleted. Providing your body does not have an insulin sensitivity or resistance problem, things should proceed well.

However, as you become older, your body's ability to regulate insulin levels may deteriorate. In order to keep up, your body will require that you work even more. That's not always feasible for it to happen. Problems will begin to occur at this time. Unnecessary glucose may be building up in your system. There's nothing you can do if your body isn't burning off what you've consumed. Most of your energy will be at its peak during these times. These, on the other hand, might leave you feeling drained and lethargic even after only a few hours. Long-term, it's pointless to experience these bursts of energization.

When your body's energy levels dip you begin to feel sluggish and need more sweets and carbohydrates. You'll naturally want more of it because that's what you originally offered your body in exchange for the energy you're receiving. As a result, you may develop harmful eating and snacking habits if you are not attentive. In order to satisfy your cravings, you may find yourself reaching for processed or artificial items, such as candy or soda. Insulin resistance isn't required to experience this. It's just a matter of how you're programming your body through the food you eat.

You're not alone if you've experienced these highs and lows in your own life. Many people feel this way on a regular basis, but they don't know how to adapt their food in a way that actually alters the pattern. Adjusting carb intake isn't adequate for most people. Mood swings and hunger pangs will set up at this point. Cutting back on carbohydrates without replacing them tells your body that you're cutting back on your energy supply. This will set off a chain reaction of resistance inside you, which will inevitably lead to frustration. End of the day, you are likely to crave your favourite junk food.

You can make sure you're getting enough fats and proteins to balance out your carb intake by following a ketogenic diet. Maintaining your energy levels should be no problem if you stick to a Keto diet according to the recommended percentages. No extreme highs or lows, just middle points that you can get to. Instead of thinking that it is the only source of energy today, your body won't make that assumption. Because of this, it will not enter a condition of overworking and then crash. Keto is all about finding a healthy balance, so if you're looking for a way to boost your energy levels, bear that in mind.

Concerns raised by those considering the transition are likely to be similar to yours. Many people fear that Keto will not be adequate for them to maintain their weight loss goals. In their minds, this means a tonne of snacking and binge-eating throughout the day, but they're startled to discover that this is actually far less of a necessity. Let go of the negative connotations associated with dieting, and you'll discover that your body undergoes a natural process of adaptation.

Make sure that you are truly committed to the change before you begin.

Although the Ketogenic diet drains your energy reserves, it replaces them with fats that are good for you. ' Many people believe that Keto is harmful for you since it seems like you're starving yourself, but that isn't how it actually works.. You are merely altering the way your body functions and the method in which it makes use of this kinetic energy. Instead of resenting you for making this choice, your body will be grateful. As a matter of fact, you'll soon discover that your body is able to dip into these additional reserves for more fuel anytime it is needed. When you give it these good fats, it will learn how to use them and how to keep them available for a long length of time.

End your afternoon slumps and feel like you have enough energy to get through any workday with this supplement. Having fewer meals during the day means you're less likely to get cranky or "hangry." As a rule, your body waits for your next meal when you're not eating. A Keto diet allows you to go about your day without feeling like you're being distracted by hunger or cravings since your body is storing this energy in reserves. Be aware that everyone's experience with the Keto diet will be unique. Retraining your body to eat less carbohydrates may take some time, depending on how much of your diet is composed of them currently. Even for the vast majority of people, this happens rather rapidly. To begin reaping the benefits of the ketogenic diet, you may have to suffer with a few days of stomach discomfort, but this should not stop you. Positive Weight Loss and a Clearer Mind

To put the science of Keto into practise in your own life, you'll likely be eager to do so after you've learned it. In the long run, with all the stated advantages, it's a long-term option for losing weight and getting your life back on track. Optimal health can only be achieved when your mind and body are in harmony. You may expect a smooth transition when you begin your Keto adventure. Even while results aren't going to come quickly with this eating plan, they will be long-lasting once you see them. Not a 10lb/week diet, this is a long-term lifestyle change. It's a way of life that keeps the pounds off for good.

There are many benefits to following a Ketogenic diet, and if you're willing to stick with it, it's a good choice.

We'll go into the specific foods you'll be consuming on the Keto diet in this part of the guide. To get you started, we've compiled a list of some of the most popular Keto-friendly dinners. New and inventive dishes, as well as alterations to tried-and-true favourites, will be at your fingertips after you've mastered the principles of healthy eating. You should not put too much pressure on yourself to come up with a detailed food plan when you first start off. This is something

TIPS   25

you can always become better at. An all-inclusive meal plan can help you get started and provide you the flexibility to try new things once you've gained the confidence to do so.

On Monday morning, I had scrambled eggs on a bed of lettuce for breakfast.

Lunch: grilled fish on a bed of spinach.

Dinner: Red cabbage slaw with pork chops

Tuesday: Sunflower seeds and a variety of nuts and seeds for snacking.

Breakfast — Coconut oil and butter coffee (Google)

Look up "bulletproof coffee recipes" for some interesting concepts.) in addition to a few cooked eggs

Brunch: Stuffed tomatoes with tuna salad

Dinner - Zucchini noodles topped with meatballs and a creamy sauce.

Mixing berries with Macadamia nuts is an excellent snack option on Wednesday.

Breakfast omelette with salsa and cheese and vegetables

lunch: sashimi and miso soup (takeout)

Roasted chicken with asparagus and mushrooms in a white wine sauce for dinner (in butter)

Breakfast: Greek yoghurt with nuts on top and an almond milk smoothie with greens and protein powder for snacks. Thursday:

An almond milk smoothie with spinach and protein powder for breakfast is ideal.

Lunch: Chicken tenders with cucumbers and goat cheese on a bed of greens.

grilled shrimp with lemon and broccoli for dinner

Eggs, cheese, and peppers cut thinly as a snack

Friday:

Fried eggs, bacon, and greens for breakfast.

Avocado on a lettuce sandwich, served with a side salad, for lunch.

A Thai peanut butter sauce drizzled over baked tofu and served with a side of cauliflower rice, broccoli, and bell peppers makes a hearty dinner.

Snacks — Walnuts, mixed berries, and celery coated in almond butter Saturday:

Baked eggs with avocado halves as a breakfast dish

Poached salmon and avocado rolls with seaweed wraps for lunch

Beef kebabs on the grill with peppers and broccoli for dinner

Kale chips and sugar-free jerky (beef or turkey) for Sunday snacking

Eggs scrambled with vegetables and salsa for breakfast

Lunch – Tuna salad served in avocado halves with mayonnaise.

Dinner — Broiled trout with butter and bok choy sautéed in butter

Dry seaweed with cheese slivers for a snack.

Chapter Three

The diet

Many of the meals in these two example Keto weeks are likely to be favourites of yours that you eat on a regular basis currently. This is a huge advantage of the Keto diet because much of the stuff you'll be consuming is likely to be familiar to you. Maintaining a Keto-friendly diet doesn't need giving up all of your favourite foods. Many times, all you have to do is eat more of the foods and meals that you already like. This week's worth of meals is meant to give you some ideas for your own weekly menu.

You may want to cook most of your meals at home if your present schedule allows for it, depending on how much time you have available. There is a wide range of choices on the menus in terms of the sources of the cuisine. In the event that takeout is already part of your daily routine, it's still a choice. Many others, on the other hand, determine that Keto is a turning point. As a result, they frequently plan their meals in advance so that they can stay on track with their diets. Takeout and restaurant meals are also options, but you should exercise extreme caution when it comes to the foods they use. Almost usually, some sort of adjustment is going to be required.

You should be aware of these possibilities since, in certain cases, dining out is the only option you have available to you. There will be occasions when you need to dine with others, whether it's a lunch date with a buddy or a work meeting away from the office. People on diets often worry that going out to eat with friends and having a good time will be replaced with sitting there without a plate of food. Keto doesn't necessitate complete abstinence from all food groups. If you're on Keto and going out to eat, the best advice is to focus on getting enough protein. You'll almost certainly find a protein-heavy meal at each restaurant you visit

After you've decided on a protein, find out what sides are included. Vegetables or dairy products may generally take the place of carbs in most recipes. Prior you deciding to skip the entrée entirely, be sure to enquire about possible replacements. Servers are more likely to provide recommendations if you tell them what you can and cannot eat. Every day, people on diets go out to eat, and most restaurants are tolerant of their needs. In the course of your keto diet, don't hesitate to ask for tweaks and alternatives. Make sure you approach your diet plan as if it were your own.

Design the procedure even more efficient for yourself if you choose to make your own Keto-friendly dinner from scratch. There are many who adore cooking every day while others simply don't have the time. You can substantially benefit from meal preparing. The amount of time you'll save when it comes to cooking is directly proportional to the amount of shopping and meal preparation you can accomplish in one day. Take note of dishes that seem fascinating and healthful while planning your meals in advance. You'll likely be able to make better judgments in the grocery shop if you know these ideas in advance.

Relax while you're preparing your meals. Knowing that you're making an investment in your health even if cooking isn't your favourite thing to do can help you persevere through the process. Prepare and store all of the food you'll need for the week, and then split it out into individual containers. Ideally, all of the food should be sorted according to meal type. ' You'll be able to heat up a serving whenever you want and take it with you wherever you go. There are plenty of Keto meal prep dishes that can be eaten either hot or cold, making them ideal for when you're away from home or the kitchen. Even your kids could be interested in your new food prep methods.

Meal planning should be done as a team effort between all members of the family, therefore this is an excellent approach to do it. There are a variety of reasons why eating healthfully might be challenging, but when presented with a variety of alternatives, it becomes much simpler. Display the dishes you've created and the ones you've grown to love for your family to see. The chances are that your family and friends will like your meals just as much as you do, even if they aren't following the Keto diet. Recipes may be added to at any time to a convenient recipe book. You'll be more likely to recall them if you keep track of them on a regular basis.

Remember that you may dine out and cook at the same time while on the keto diet. The most important thing is to take a look at your lifestyle and existing routine and see what works for you. It's possible to get started with

THE DIET   29

meal planning even if you just have a few days to spare, so give it a try. When it comes to eating, there should be no need for a one-size-fits-all approach. Attention to one's own body is the key. If you find that eating out saps your energy, it's possible that you're not receiving enough nutrients. Cooking your own meals is the greatest method to ensure that you are providing your body with the nutrients it needs. When you are able to listen to your body, you will always know what you need to do the next time.

The following is a critical point to keep in mind

The "Keto flu" can strike if you aren't vigilant, so exercise caution. You may experience this if you go right into the Keto diet without a gradual adjustment period. One of the most common symptoms is a flu-like illness, which occurs when the body adjusts to a die without carbohydrates. Headaches, constipation, and nausea are some of the most common manifestations. Despite the fact that many individuals are able to effectively transition into the diet without experiencing any of these symptoms, you may have to cope with them for a short amount of time. When it comes to avoiding the Keto flu, staying hydrated is one of the most important steps. When you're dehydrated, your body is losing minerals it needs to function properly. Try sugar-free electrolyte drinks if water isn't enough to rehydrate you.

It's also vital to bear in mind any preexisting problems. For those with pancreas, liver, thyroid, or gallbladder issues the Keto diet is inappropriate for them. Low blood pressure and nutritional inadequacies might result if you don't eat a well-balanced diet. Taking a multivitamin on a daily basis might help you avoid this. The most essential thing to remember while embarking on a diet is to avoid intense activity. It is critical that you give your body time to adapt to the Ketogenic diet before overworking it.

Dietary Appetite Regulator

When starting the Keto diet, it's critical to have a strategy in place for managing your hunger. Your body may overreact and overeat if you make any modifications to your typical eating habits. The consequences of this on your health and nutrition might be dire if it occurs regularly. You need to be self-disciplined to stick to any diet plan, no matter how stringent or loose it is. Your Keto diet and lifestyle are now complete, and you need to keep them in mind at all times. It's normal for your body to be pleased while you're not eating or snacking. That want to binge on junk food or wish you had more food isn't something you should be experiencing. Despite the fact that Keto leads your body into thinking it's in "starvation mode," you shouldn't feel this way on the outside.

Being aware of these warning signs will help keep you on track when on a Keto diet. As a general rule, it isn't intended to feel awful or be difficult to sustain. No part of your body should ever feel worse than it did before. Constipation and stomach discomfort are common side effects of the keto diet. However, there should be no long-term pain in your body. There could be a problem with your food plan if this is happening, so it's time to take a closer look at it. Don't allow yourself to succumb to the idea that this awful sensation is a permanent part of your life.

If you're always hungry in between meals, it's possible that you need to up your snacking game. Because the Keto diet does not need careful calorie control, snacking is not considered "cheating." Snacks aren't a terrible thing if you need them to keep you going between meals. Transitioning from one diet to another might cause some discomfort. The convenience of meal preparing your snacks means that you'll always have something to satisfy a hunger. You will be less inclined to deviate from your diet plan if you only have nutritious and Keto-friendly snacks available to you. Keeping your snacks divided into manageable servings is a great method to keep track of how much you're eating at any one time.

Working exercise can be a part of your weekly routine or a part of your everyday routine, depending on your schedule. Think about the amount of energy you expend when you get up and move, no matter how often you do. In general, it's not a smart idea to work out when you're starving. As soon as you begin your workout, you may feel dizzy or sick to your stomach. Make an effort to consume light food and drink plenty of fluids prior to and throughout your workout. Afterwards, you'll need to refill your body's energy stores. Your body will be able to create greater muscle mass if you eat protein within 30 minutes of exercising. Adding a scoop of protein powder to your pre- or post-workout smoothie might provide the extra push you need. You only need to keep track of your protein consumption percentages to avoid overdoing it. Inflammation levels are reduced.

Keto has anti-inflammatory properties due to its detoxifying properties. As a result, your body is able to rid itself of all that sugar instead of storing it. Your body will automatically reduce the amount of inflammation it clings onto once you've gotten rid of these extra glucose reserves. Inflammation may lead to a slew of health issues, and as a woman in her fifties, this is especially true. Inflamed joints make it difficult to do numerous everyday tasks. If your joints are inflamed, you will have difficulty doing anything, from walking to sitting in

THE DIET 31

a car for extended periods of time. It's all about your diet, because you know that the items on the Keto diet help to reduce inflammation.

When you wake up in the morning, you'll notice a difference in your levels of inflammation since Keto is effectively managing them. Jumping out of bed and getting moving soon is never a smart idea, but when you are inflamed, there is no other choice. Your body will have an easier time adjusting to being awake if the burning and stiffness are alleviated. Your alarm clock should wake you up automatically, so you don't have to repeatedly press the snooze button. Start your day on the right foot by waking up when you're supposed to, rather than snoozing the alarm.

If you've ever had inflammation, you've probably observed that sitting or standing for lengthy periods of time makes it worse. As a result, for the majority of us, the inflammatory response is at its most severe when we are working. In some cases, anti-inflammatory drugs are all that's needed to alleviate the discomfort, but this isn't always the case. If you don't have to, becoming reliant on medicine is not a pleasant experience. When it comes to an inflamed body, this is why Keto might be beneficial. Instead of popping a pill, try modifying your diet to reduce inflammation. As long as you are adhering to your Keto diet, the detoxification process will begin immediately. Your inflammation should be reduced as a result of this treatment.

Towards the end of the day, your body has a natural tendency to swell up and get irritated, and this tendency increases. Because you may be exhausted, but your inflammation is keeping you awake with restless leg syndrome or neck and back discomfort, this may be really inconvenient. Rather of pondering your supper choices, you've probably grabbed for a prescription in the past.

When you think of your body as a machine, you'll be better able to stick to your Keto diet. When you consider how much better you'll feel on Keto, it should be worth it to adhere to the diet despite the temptations that lurk around every turn.

Age-related inflammation is normal. Preventative actions will assist you in the long term, even if you can't avoid it entirely. The Keto diet might be viewed as a prophylactic measure. For the most part, you can keep your physical health in check with this eating plan, which is a terrific method to lose weight. The diet you're on should allow you to look as well as feel good about yourself. When it comes to going on the keto diet, it's not just about looking good. Even if you've been unwell for a long time, you can get your health back on track with this programme. No time is ever too late to change for the better. This is an unfortunate but widely held erroneous belief among many people.

You'll be surprised at how much simpler your daily tasks become once your body stops resting in an inflammatory state. A good night's sleep might begin with a less inflamed body, which can allow you to sleep better. As a result, you'll be able to get out of bed earlier and accomplish more in the morning. A well-rested body is a powerful tool for achieving a variety of goals. If you overwork yourself and then don't eat enough to compensate, you'll always be tired and depressed.

It's easier to work out when there's less inflammation in the body. The need of regular physical exercise for women over 50 cannot be overstated, even if you don't follow a strict bodybuilding plan. Your body is meant to be in motion, not sedentary, so it's important to maintain it that way. Your metabolism will be boosted and your energy levels will rise as a result of the Keto diet. Everything in your body is interconnected, even if it doesn't appear that way at first. In general, less inflammation equates to less strain. You should keep a journal of how you feel before and after starting the Keto diet. What you discover is sure to astound you. Plus, there aren't any cheap tricks to be found. Keto is a diet that works in concert with your body, not against it.

For a clean mind, eat clean food.

What does the word "clean eating" mean in the context of your new Keto way of life? Eat natural, whole foods wherever feasible as a cornerstone of clean eating. Preservative- and additive-laden packaged foods are discouraged in the clean eating movement, which advocates the use of only fresh, unadulterated ingredients. Eating clean may take some time and effort for individuals who aren't used to it, but the benefits far outweigh the inconveniences. In the long run, the less room your body has for bad carbs and fats, the better. Clean eating and digestion go hand in hand.

You'll also be able to think more clearly as a result of this.

If you aren't currently following a clean diet, you may be depriving your body of essential nutrients. Natural meals are the only ones that provide the ideal ratio of nutrients for optimal physiological function. Canned and preserved vegetables are not nearly as nutritious as fresh ones, even if you consume them often. You can improve your health and the environment by making tiny improvements like these. The organic-only grocery shop isn't necessary, but you may start by focusing on these tiny aspects.

THE DIET   33

While on a keto diet, you are urged to eat meals that are low in carbohydrates and high in protein. A straightforwa d approach is required for preparing your meats and veggies. These are the items that you will use to flavour the rest of the cuisine, with the occasional ad ition of butter or dairy products. Make sure the meat you buy is always fresh. L's best to utilise it right away rather than risk it going bad in your freezer because you forgot to label it. Fresh veggies are an excellent choice for the Keto diet. Because the fresher options taste better and provide more nutrition, it coesn't make sense to go for the canned kind. If you can't get your hands on fresh vegetables, frozen vegetables are a better alternative than canned ones.

Eating clean has the added benefit of providing you with access to a wealth of information. The Keto diet necessitates that you become intimately familiar with the ingredients you're ingesting. When you follow a clean diet, you'll always be aware of how much protein, fat, and carbohydrate you're consuming. You'll benefit from knowing this knowledge in general as well as for staying on track with your Keto diet. Knowing what you're consuming and how it affects your body is essential.

Cleaning up one's diet also entails sourcing ingredients as locally as possible. Use locally sourced ingredients to help smaller farms while also cutting down on your carbon impact. Because mass-producing food requires a lot of resources, it makes more sense to use locally accessible resources. Because the world's food supply is finite, making better food choices now will have a positive impact on the planet's food supply in the future. Make an effort to visit local farmer's markets as often as you can. You may be able to find a few in your immediate vicinity. Since many of these items aren't normally found in supermarkets, you may find new delicacies that you hadn't previously had access to

Eating clean has been shown to have mental health benefits, as well. This is feasible due to the fact that consuming healthy foods may have a positive effect on one's mental state. Your body will benefit greatly from a diet high in whole foods. Your physical well-being will improve, but so will your emotional well-being. As a result, your outlook and outlook on life will be improved. Even your mind seems to undergo the same purification process as your physical body. You'll find that you're more effective in social situations and at work when your thinking is more clear. As you go about your daily business, you'll keep your mental faculties at their sharpest.

Clean eating, on the other hand, is a more enjoyable experience. You'd probably devour your favourite fast food burger in a jiffy if you grabbed one. Imagine a salad that includes all of your favourite foods. Which one would you have to eat more of? Due to the time it takes to eat it, the salad would be the best option. Is eating fast food always a good idea? Our physical health is at risk if we put too much emphasis on eating quickly. Digesting food more easily is made easier by allowing ourselves to relish the experience of eating. Slowing down your metabolism allows your body to better absorb the food you're ingesting. Think about what your body needs before you eat, rather than merely consuming food to fill yourself up. Consider what sort of fuel you can offer yourself so that you may be the best version of yourself imaginable. If you had slowed down, you'll be thankful for it.

Foods to Maintain a Stable Blood Sugar Leve.

The only thing on your mind when you eat is satiating your hunger. Despite the fact that this is a significant component of eating, it is not the sole one. Older people have a harder time keeping their blood sugar levels constant. This is a normal occurrence, and you have no control over it. If you don't make an attempt to control it, the ageing process isn't very forgiving. As your body ages, you won't be able to feel your best since you'll be eating things that aren't appropriately nourishing it. You should eat in order to maintain a stable level of energy by regulating your blood sugar levels. It should be able to satisfy your hunger and refill your supply. You'll acquire one of these side effects if you consume a lot of fast food. However, being satisfied does not equate to being in good health.

Think about the last time you ate and how full you felt afterward. Did you wish you hadn't eaten so much food because you were so full? What did you think of the dinner as a whole? Did you feel peckish again shortly after your meal? Using the answers to these questions, you may get an idea of how nutritious your diet is. Even if your meals are made with healthy components, this does not imply that you are eating in the healthiest manner. The Keto diet teaches you to rethink your eating habits. It promotes healthy eating by allowing you to consume large, filling meals. You should be able to maintain a healthy lifestyle on this diet.

By now, you've become familiar with the link between carbohydrates and blood sugar. To maintain your body in tiptop shape while on the Keto diet, you'll want to understand how the diet works to reduce excess sugar. Remember that Keto is meant to help you regulate your blood sugar levels, rather

THE DIET   35

than completely eradicate them. This glucose is essential for our survival. Keto-friendly foods aren't meant to be completely eliminated from your diet. Instead, you're looking for a healthier, more harmonious state of being. There will be health issues if you have too much or too little of something your body naturally produces. Keeping to a strict Keto diet plan is essential for this reason. So that you don't drain your body's resources, they maintain you healthy and functional.

Remember, you're doing this for your long-term health and well-being, not for quick weight loss. While on the diet, avoid depriving yourself of anything; otherwise, it won't work. Overcompensation is a natural response to a shortage of something in your body. When it needs to focus on this instead of focusing on getting into a state of ketosis, then your body is going to be missing the goal when it comes to eating Keto. This is why many individuals think that eating Keto involves preparation. By reading this guide, you are taking the steps essential that you need in order to get started the proper way. When you are informed on the diet to the best of your abilities, you will be better able to follow it appropriately.

If you are overly restricted while on the Keto diet, this might lead your body to become insulin sensitive. This happens when the body stops manufacturing as much glucose, thereby creating less insulin. Keep in mind that you don't have to entirely give up carbohydrates on any of the various Keto diets. While you are going to be eating a fraction of the quantity that you formerly ate, you are still going to be receiving some in your system in order to prevent these health risks. A lot of individuals who are sceptical about the Keto diet tend to assume that the body is going to run into these difficulties when attempting to consume fewer carbohydrates. Balance is key when it comes to dieting and as long as you are following the suggested carb consumption, then you should be just fine.

On the other end of the diet, if you do not follow it well enough, then your body isn't going to start creating and storing less glucose. This frequently happens when people try to follow the diet, but do not have the resolve to maintain going. Keto might potentially be more harmful to your health than not beginning at all. If you are going to be doing things partly, then you should hold off until you feel that you are ready to completely commit to the diet. You cannot expect to follow some of the guidelines yet obtain the same wonderful outcomes and benefits. Being realistic with your approach is going to save you from the frustration and the inconvenience of not getting the results that you are anticipating.

Stop and take a breather if you feel like you're losing track of what you should be consuming. Think about the benefits of the Keto diet and utilise them as motivation in order to maintain eating appropriately. It is normal to have cravings at different times of the week. You'll be able to maintain your concentration if you can recognise your feelings without giving in to them. A change in your blood sugar levels may convey a message to your brain that you need sugar. Know that this is only a cry for help, but that your body is going to shift on its own in order to start burning energy from fats instead. Remember why you started the Keto diet in the first place and eat foods high in healthy fats and protein to keep yourself calm.

For a Powerful Life, Eat a Clean Diet.

In terms of detoxifying, the Keto diet is an excellent choice. Detoxing doesn't need being hungry and without food. In other words, you're allowing your body to benefit from the healthiest, most natural foods possible. This relates to our prior discussion on healthy living, but it merits a more in-depth look.

Consider natural while making your meal selections; if you have trouble pronouncing the ingredients, it's probably best to avoid it. Despite the fact that several chemicals are in place to keep our food fresh, they should not be ingested on a daily basis. Even while occasional use of processed foods poses no immediate threat, your body will become accustomed to them over time. As a result, adopting a healthy eating regimen becomes more difficult.

As long as there are no chemicals in your food, your body is able to utilise all of it. Your body will be able to begin the process of turning fats into energy instead of needing to go through what is nutritious and what isn't, and what has to be filtered or cleansed by your liver. It will have a clear and defined purpose. The goal of the Keto diet is to assist your body achieve this clarity. As a result, you can be confident that everything you consume has a specific function and intended usage in mind because it does not include any extraneous substances. When you give your body these natural components to operate with, it will know exactly what to do.

Everyone may get the benefits of a food detox, according to recent studies. Even if it isn't a long-term solution, committing to a clean eating regimen for a few weeks can do wonders for your body's internal clock. With the Ketogenic diet, you don't have to adhere to a rigorous diet to get the advantages of a cleanse. Juice cleanses are the most common method of detox, but this isn't the only one. There are several layers to the process, just like in any other

THE DIET   37

endeavour. It's possible to cleanse your body while still eating as much as you normally do.

While on the Keto diet, you'll have to deal with a lot of temptation. If you work hard enough, you'll be able to handle them better and better as time goes on. Despite popular belief, the urges to binge do lessen with time. The craving for sugar will be forgotten once your body is able to rid itself of it completely. For a short time, you may experience cravings for sugar, but as time passes, your body will start to crave other things. You may notice a shift in your desire for sweets to desire protein. Due to the misconception that their bodies will want sweets the entire time, many people avoid the keto diet. These first desires may be overcome and you'll discover that it's far easier than you believe to keep these urges under check.

Changing poor habits to good ones and adjusting your perspective from negative to positive is all that is required to achieve success. Whenever we make a lifestyle change, this is a normal shift, and we're built to reject it. So, let's look at a few approaches to dealing with this extremely prevalent problem.

Adapting Your Lifestyle and Attitude to Affect Your Physical Health

Dieting involves adhering to a set of rules. When you already have a set of rules in place, the transition from one to the other is a lengthy one. Think of your Keto diet as a temporary shift in your lifestyle, rather than a permanent one. Getting started on the diet will be easier if you approach it with the perspective that it is a positive and healthy change. Knowing what to eat and how you should feel will allow you to compare how you really feel to how the diet is intended to make you feel. With this method, you don't feel like you have to entirely give up control over your nutrition.

Among our many flaws are our negative habits, many of which are dietary in nature. Convenience is a powerful motivator in today's world, making it simple to fall into bad habits. In a pinch, you may choose to order takeout rather than cook a dinner for yourself because of the ingrained belief that it is quicker and less time-consuming. Even if it's quicker, the quality of the food you're consuming is probably suffering as a result of your haste. Cooking for one's self doesn't necessitate much more work in most cases. Fast food and food delivery services have become so commonplace that it's little wonder you'd prefer to have someone else prepare your meals for you.

You may save money by using some of these services, but you have no way of knowing what you are consuming. To your knowledge, you do not know where the components come from or how they were created. All of these factors contribute to your general well-being, but they become even more critical as you get older. In this day and age, it is more important than ever to pay attention to where your food comes from. Let others determine what is best for your body when you let these decisions fall out of your hands. Junk food addiction is so strong that even when you feel lethargic, your body will convince you that you must keep eating this way.

Focuses on what you are already doing and how you can improve it for your own health. It's difficult, but not impossible, to modify your behaviours. Real results may be achieved as long as you have the will and determination to keep going. A poor habit can take years to develop, so if you don't see a difference right away, don't worry. Even if this stage takes some time, your ultimate aim of improving your health will be closer each time you put in the effort. Remember that this is something you're doing only for yourself. When things get tough, remember how good you feel when you eat healthy, whole foods. This will help you get back on track when things get tough.

Changes to Be Made: A Step-by-Step Guide

When you're requested to modify your eating habits, it's a lot easier said than done. Even if you have a clear vision of the final product, getting there might be a challenge. Breaking this component down into daily stages is the key. Change is difficult, and it won't happen overnight. It takes time for the body and the mind to adapt to the new and preferable alterations. Step one is already done if you can make a daily commitment to working on these behaviours. You'll see actual results if you're dedicated to the cause. You may expect the same consequences if you're only 50% engaged in success.

Breakfast is the first meal of the day.

If you want to make changes to the way you eat, you may do it one meal at a time. Consider the way you begin each day. A good question is: Do you have breakfast or wait until lunch instead? For those who skip breakfast, but then graze heavily until lunch, this might lead to weight gain. Even if you do have breakfast, the high sugar and carbohydrate content may have detrimental consequences. Breakfast is the most important meal of the day since it sets the tone for the rest of the day. The purpose of breakfast is to provide you with energy to get you through the morning and into the afternoon when you are able to sit down and eat lunch. Breakfast is often considered to be the most essential meal of the day, as you may already be aware.

THE DIET   39

In the morning, even if you don't feel like you're hungry, try to eat something nutritious. It's not necessary to have a large breakfast, but getting some protein into your system before you begin your day will make a significant impact. Breakfasts on the ketogenic diet can be as small or as large as you choose. A lot of people wake up feeling a little hungry, but that's perfectly OK. At the very least, try to make smoothies a regular part of your diet so that you have something to eat. You should notice an increase in your energy levels after a week of doing this. At the start of the day, you'll be able to concentrate better.

Stay hydrated.

Keep an eye on how much water you're consuming during the day. Even if you're on a strict diet, water is always the healthiest choice of beverage. You should drink as much water as possible when on the keto diet. When you're properly hydrated, your entire body functions better. Whenever you start to feel hungry, drinking a glass of water will fill you up and provide you energy. In spite of the fact that drinking water isn't going to make you feel full, it may keep you hydrated and help you feel wonderful between meals. Staying hydrated is critical while engaging in any strenuous activity. The body's moisture needs increase as we get older. Hydrate with electrolytes if you begin to get the "keto flu" (sugar-free).

Limit your intake of sweetened beverages.

If you don't drink water, keep an eye on the amount of sugar in your beverage of choice. Even fresh fruit juices might have a lot of natural sugars in them. You'll have to be careful with your choices if you're following the Keto diet, which emphasises avoiding sugar. You don't have to worry about how much sugar you're eating when you drink water. High fructose corn syrup-laden drinks and juices are difficult for many individuals to give up. The more familiar something is to you, the more difficult it is to let it go of it. If you're having a hard time getting yourself to drink water, you may want to experiment with natural flavourings. Fruits may be used to infuse water to give it an extra taste boost.

Lunches That Are Good For You

Over lunch, brainstorm about how you may improve things. People often overlook the importance of how quickly they eat their meals, which can have a significant impact on their health. Lunch is frequently had during a scheduled break at work or elsewhere. If you find yourself in the same predicament, remember that you don't have to rush through lunch. Trying to eat healthily might lead to overeating or eating too much of the wrong item. Lunchtime is a great time to employ meal planning because you'll already have a well-balanced meal prepared for you. Bring your lunch to work if you haven't done so yet.

A Ketogenic Diet Outside of the House

As you know, the Keto diet allows you to eat out at least a couple times over the course of your day. Since the regulations will remain the same, it is up to you to suggest modifications as needed. Request substitutes if a dish includes carbohydrates. Many people understand what the Ketogenic diet entails when you tell them you're following it. However, if you're attempting to stick to a certain diet, it's up to you to make sure that people who will be preparing your meals know what you're eating. There should be no misunderstanding regarding the necessity of avoiding carbohydrates by emphasising that fats and dairy products are the only acceptable food choices.

When you're out to eat, don't be hesitant to voice your opinions. This is the most common reason why diets fail, namely because making adjustments is perceived as an inconvenience. If you're serious about following a Ketogenic diet, you'll want to keep a close eye on your food intake. Because no one else is going to do it for you, sticking to the rules is all the more of a success. When eating out, be rigorous with yourself even if Keto isn't a restrictive diet. Being in the company of friends or family members might be enticing at times. As long as they're eating what you'd like to be eating, you're more likely to believe that you can, too. Keep in mind that if you make one mistake, your body may not be able to enter ketosis. As a result, the Keto diet won't be as effective as it once was.

In no way can this be seen as a criticism of dining with others. Even if temptations abound, it is possible to maintain a Keto diet and yet have a good time during a group meal. In order to avoid the items that you are attempting to avoid, explain to your family and friends what the diet consists of and why. As a result, you have a better chance of forgetting about and not needing carbohydrates and sweets when they aren't available. There are several benefits to eating with others, including an increase in morale. You'll have more fun dining when you put your attention on the people you're with than than the food you're not allowed to consume. Strategic Meal Scheduling

Be aware that you'll need some time to eat and digest. It is important to avoid eating too close to bedtime while having a meal that is traditionally consumed at home. As a result of the high meat content of the Keto diet, eating late at night might make you feel sluggish and lethargic. Try to keep to a supper hour

THE DIET   41

that you've chosen. This will train your digestive system to digest food at a certain rate and establish a regular eating schedule for you. On the Keto diet, getting into these habits is a terrific way to keep yourself in check. It's best to start with a healthy diet and then ease into more strenuous exercises. You should never eat before going to sleep.. An unsettled stomach and the belief that you've finished digesting can be caused by this. As a result, you're more than likely going to have trouble sleeping or feeling calm.

Snacking on Keto

Make a shift in your thinking about snacking. If you have any unfavourable feelings about snacking while on the Keto diet, you should realise that this is not required. It's not only possible to make your own Keto snacks, but nibbling is also an excellent strategy to get you through the day. To help your body adapt, you may find yourself snacking more frequently than ever before. It's all right! Your diet is safe as long as you have a wide variety of healthy foods accessible. Unlike a meal, a snack isn't going to completely fill you up, but it should suffice until you can eat something more substantial. Bring a few snacks with you if you're going to be out from home for an extended period of time. You won't be tempted to buy bad meal this way.

Preparing Meals

In your kitchen, keep a recipe book. You'll be able to find all of your favourite Keto-friendly recipes here. If you ever find yourself scrambling to put together a dinner or need inspiration for meal planning, this list will come in handy. Always keep an eye out for new recipes you'd like to experiment with. Your recipe book should be organised according to what you've tried and liked, as well as what you want to attempt in the future. It's possible to organise them by meal type or culinary style if you so like. This is an area where you have a lot of creative leeway, so go ahead and play with with it as much as you like! You'll notice a difference in the quality of your meals when you get more comfortable in the kitchen.

At a Meal at a Time: Creating New Habits.

In spite of their simplicity, these tips will inspire you to make significant improvements. As with the Keto diet, you may continue to make modifications in your regular routine to optimise your nutrition. It's not always easy to get into a better frame of mind, but the more you do it, the more natural it will become. While away from home, you will be able to demonstrate to yourself that you can maintain a healthy diet and resist the need to overindulge. It's always possible to return to a solid foundation if you can maintain it. In order to keep yourself motivated, constantly remind yourself of how you are improving your whole well-being, both physically and mentally.

When practising intermittent fasting, a person should incorporate the following items into their daily diet and eating periods in order to keep their insulin levels under control:

A significant amount of omega-3 fats may be found in fatty fish such as herring, salmon, sardines, mackerel, and anchovies. [Citation needed] In addition to being beneficial for one's blood sugar levels, eating fatty fish may also reduce one's chance of developing cardiovascular disease. In addition to these benefits, it has been shown to reduce inflammatory indicators in the body and improve cognitive function.

Eggs are not only one of the finest meals to eat to lower insulin levels, but they are also one of the best foods to consume if you want to feel fuller for a longer period of time after eating them. They are also beneficial for lowering the risk of developing cardiovascular disease because they provide fuel for the muscles, reduce insulin resistance, and bring inflammatory indicators to lower levels.

Greek yoghurt is another another meal that aids in lowering the levels of sugar in the blood. It is also a highly adaptable meal that may be used in lieu of mayonnaise in many other applications. You may use it to thicken smoothies, eat it as a meal on its own, enjoy it as a dessert topped with berries, or use it as a replacement for ice cream.

When it comes to fruits that are high in health benefits, strawberries are at the top of the list. They have a very high concentration of antioxidants, particularly anthocyanin, which is the pigment responsible for their distinctive hue. Anthocyanin has been shown to lessen the chance of developing heart disease, as well as reducing cholesterol and blood sugar levels after a meal.

Nuts are a good source of fibre. As a result of their low digestible carb content, they are an excellent choice for those watching their carbohydrate intake. There are, on the other hand, certain nuts that are a

somewhat more carbohydrates than the others. However, a person ought to incorporate cashews, Brazil nuts, hazelnuts, almonds, pistachios, walnuts, and pecans into their diet.

THE DIET   43

Even if a person does not have diabetes or any other condition that requires them to monitor or regulate their blood sugar, they should still make an effort to include turmeric in their diet. In addition to acting as a natural component in the regulation of insulin levels, it possesses qualities that make it effective in combating cancer and lowers the chance of developing heart disease.

Seeds, such as flax seeds, include a high amount of fibre, which can assist in lowering insulin levels. Chia seeds are another excellent seed source that are full of fibre and other components that not only lower insulin levels but also lower the risk of heart disease and cancer. Chia seeds help reduce the risk of diabetes.

Vegetables like spinach, lettuce, and kale that are dark green and leafy, such as aid to manage insulin levels while also lowering the chance of developing heart disease. Additionally, they are jam-packed with vitamins and other essential elements that the body need, particularly when it is fasting.

Garlic is not only used to enhance the flavour of food; it also possesses a variety of beneficial benefits for one's health. The ability to help manage insulin levels, the ability to fight cancer, and the ability to reduce the risk of heart disease are some of these benefits.

Because cinnamon offers so many benefits, it need to be incorporated into a person's regular eating routine in some way. One notable advantage is that it reduces the amount of insulin that is released into the bloodstream after meals.

The meal known as squash is one that does not receive as much attention as it should. All varieties of squash, including winter squash (butternut, pumpkin, and zucchini), as well as summer squash (zucchini, patty pan, and others), can help reduce insulin levels and obesity.

Another food that a significant number of individuals find very unappealing is broccoli. They choose going for the cauliflower instead. While cauliflower does have its advantages, broccoli is a carbohydrate that is very simple to digest and provides vitamin C in addition to a variety of other essential elements and vitamins.

Cleansing Foods That Boost Your Energy and Vitality

There are several meals that can assist in the process of detoxifying the body. If a person is attempting to detox, there are some kinds of food they should stay away from.

Some examples of foods to avoid include:

Because dairy products are acidic, they can slow down the detoxification process. This is because dairy products can cause cells to stop working as they should, which can slow down the detoxification process.

Because of its poisonous nature and negative impact on the liver, one should avoid drinking alcohol at all costs. Alcohol use lowers levels of magnesium and zinc, both of which are essential for the detoxification process.

Meat takes a long time to digest and encourages the growth of germs in the digestive tract since it does not break down very quickly. The bacteria in question is not of the beneficial variety either. Because meat is difficult for the body to digest, the process of breaking it down takes more time than usual, which in turn slows down the digestive process.

Caffeine is another dangerous substance since it is known to raise levels of toxicity within the body.

Additionally, salt is not great for the body and has been shown to cause an increase in blood pressure in certain people. A significant amount of damage may be caused by high blood pressure, and it also raises the chance of having a stroke. Because it slows down the natural activity of cells, it is also not beneficial for detoxification.

Sugar, particularly processed sugar, should be avoided at all costs. Even brown sugar that is not made from organic sugar cane has been refined. It also causes a conflict with the beneficial bacteria that are normally found in a person's stomach, which can be harmful to the detoxification process. Sugar may provide a person with an immediate surge of energy, but that burst of energy can fade very fast, leaving you feeling exhausted after consuming it. In addition to this, it has a high potential for addiction since it causes the body to seek a sugar rush.

Stay away from foods that are pre-packaged and foods that have artificial colours or tastes. It is also important to steer clear of foods that have a high sodium content or are high in saturated fat.

Some examples of foods that might help you cleanse and give you more energy are as follows:

Veggies; if you can locate organic vegetables, do so, and select fresh vegetables over frozen ones whenever possible.

THE DIET   45

Berries contain a high concentration of antioxidants. Always go for fresh berries over their dried counterparts. However, frozen berries taste just as wonderful provided that they do not include any added sugar and have a minimal or nonexistent amount of preservatives.

Whole grains include a significant amount of fibre, which not only helps with digestion but also keeps you feeling full for a longer period of time.

The majority of fruits provide a significant amount of sugar in their natural form. Not only do they help in the detoxification process, but they also help to stave off cravings for sugary foods. In addition to that, they are loaded with essential vitamins and minerals.

In addition to being an excellent source of protein, nuts and seeds also contribute to better detoxification. They also include a wide variety of beneficial elements. They also include fat-soluble vitamins, which are essential nutrients for keeping the brain functioning properly.

Ideas for a Healthy Lunch

To avoid mid-morning hunger and to carry you through the remainder of the day, lunch is essential. In general, this is the best time of the day to consume a substantial lunch. After lunch, you'll be more likely to burn off most of your food since you'll have to keep going until dinner.

Non-Limited Calorie Fasting

Typically, this is done in the evening and into the early hours of the next day. As a result, your regular eating window would begin at around 11 o'clock in the morning. Non-fasting healthy lunch ideas may be found under the non-fasting healthy ideas section. Reduce your caloric intake to maintain a healthy weight and digestive system. Rather of chowing down on a significant amount of food after a fast, sip a few glasses of water first. You'll be able to eat this and then proceed with your dinner preparation.

calorie-restricted fasting (200 to 250 Calories)

On days when you're trying to watch your caloric intake, these lunch options are perfect because they're all under 250 calories.

With grilled hake beets, ginger, and spring onion

1 piece of grilled hake

A quarter cup of raw beets shredded

2 tablespoons freshly shredded ginger root

A handful of finely sliced spring onions

1-teaspoon chilli powder

black pepper and low-sodium salt to taste

Grill is ready to go. Prepare low-sodium salt and black pepper to taste for the hake steaks, and then sprinkle with chilli spice. Place on the grill and cook for 10 to 15 minutes, or until the steak is almost done. To ensure consistent cooking, rotate the steak halfway through cooking. Shred ginger root and spring onion and sprinkle on top. After 5 to 8 minutes, put the dish back on the grill. Fresh beets are a delicious addition to the meal after it has been taken off the grill.

Smoothie with Avocado, Chocolate, and Golden Syrup - 171 Calories

a quarter of an avocado

a quarter of a banana

• 1 cup of water that has been purified

Ice cubes, about 12 cups

A single heaping tablespoon of curcumin

1 tbsp. organic raw cocoa butter

One teaspoon of vanilla essence.

Blend all of the ingredients together until smooth. Add ice cubes if the smoothie is too thin.

A Kale Wrapped Kale Salad - 223 Calories

14 avocado, cut into cubes

Grated grilled chicken breast (about 14 cup)

2 big kale leaves, roughly chopped

This recipe calls for one tablespoon of cottage cheese.

THE DIET 47

black pepper and low-sodium salt to taste

In a large bowl, combine the cottage cheese, salt, and pepper. Combine the cottage cheese with the chicken and avocado. Kale leaves should be washed and patted dry before being stacked one on top of the other. The shredded chicken, avocado, and cottage cheese should all be placed on top of one another in the centre of a leaf of kale. Wrap the leaves around the mixture and savour the flavour. If you like, you may make three smaller wraps.

Zucchini Boats with Chicken Liver Stuffing - 198 Calories

2 medium-sized squashes

cooked chicken livers-4 tablespoons

2 tbsp of parmesan

14 cups mixed salad greens, chopped

One tablespoon of pine nuts

4 cherry tomatoes, cut in half

(about 1 tablespoon)

2 tablespoons of pomegranate seeds

3 tbsp balsamic wine vinegar

black pepper and low-sodium salt to taste

Grill is ready to go. Cut the zucchini in half lengthwise, creating two boats. Make a hole in the centre of each boat (but don't cut through the zucchini) with a paring knife. Set aside the zucchini flesh that has been taken off. Divvy up the cooked chicken livers among the zucchini halves, making sure they're properly distributed throughout each one. Season the chicken livers with salt and pepper and top with parmesan cheese. Grill the zucchini boats for 8 to 10 minutes, or until they are tender.

In a large salad bowl, combine the remaining ingredients and sauté the zucchini while adding the balsamic vinegar to taste. Make a salad using the excess zucchini you removed from the centre of the boat (chop into cubes). Season to taste with salt and pepper. Serve the zucchini boats with the salad when they've finished cooking.

Slices of Eggplant Jalapeno and Prawn Pizza have 219 Calories.

▯ 1 large eggplant

Jalapenos, about two tablespoons

▯ 6 cleaned, grilled king prawns

▯ 1 tbsp organic unsweetened tomato paste

1 tbsp shredded mozzarella

1 tbsp of parmesan

Pre-heat the oven to 340°F Cut the eggplant into long, thin slices after peeling it (not too thin). Each slice should have tomato paste on one side. Shredded mozzarella can be sprinkled on top of the tomato paste. Place the prawns and jalapeño peppers on top of the tomato paste and chop them up. Give each pizza slice a generous dusting of parmesan cheese. Bake in a preheated oven at 350 degrees Fahrenheit for approximately 30 minutes, or until a toothpick inserted into the centre comes out clean.

Ideas for a Healthy Lunch on a Regular Day (500 Calories and Under)

baked potato with tuna and chunky cottage cheese, green salad on the side —

caloric intake: 383

The salt has been removed from one can of tuna in water.

two heaping spoonfuls of crumbly fat-free plain yoghurt

1 medium-sized Idaho potato for baking

14 cups mixed salad greens, chopped

One-quarter of a cucumber diced.

14 a sliced green pepper

pumpkin seeds, about two heaping tablespoons

This recipe calls for 2 tbsp of fresh basil.

3-teaspoon balsamic vinegar, organic

THE DIET   49

black pepper and low-sodium salt to taste

Mix the cottage cheese with the tuna and season with salt and pepper. Scoop out the centre of a baked potato, and then combine it with the tuna mixture. The tuna mixture should be placed in the centre of the cooked potato.. Salad ingredients should be tossed together (salad leaves, cucumber, bell pepper, pumpkin seeds, and fresh basil). Serve with the baked potato and season with salt and pepper to taste. Drizzle with balsamic vinegar.

Tomato Pita with Muscles, Lettuce and Capers - 423 Calories

The contents of one can of drained muscles

1/4 cup shredded fresh lettuce

1 pita bread of whole wheat

3 capers, minced

Chopped up a half of a tomato

4 chopped spring onions

One-quarter of a cucumber sliced.

4 tsp. cottage cheese, smooth

1 tsp of Dijon mustard

One-fourth teaspoon of cayenne pepper.

Add the cottage cheese, Dijon mustard, and cayenne pepper to a bowl and mix thoroughly. Toast the pita by cutting a slit in the top and flipping it over once it's golden brown. Combine the meat, lettuce, capers, tomatoes, onions, and cucumber in a large bowl. Combine the mayonnaise and Dijon mustard in a separate bowl and whisk until smooth. Snack on the muscle combination while it's still warm in a pita pocket.

A sandwich of toasted chicken with a spicy English mustard mayo - 464

Calories

2 whole wheat bread slices

Chicken breast shredded into 12 cup

> 1 tbsp low-fat sour cream

1 teaspoon of spicy English mustard

1 cup of roasted chips

• 2 tbsp. unsweetened margarine

Spice up the chips in the oven with Cajun seasonings if desired. Mayonnaise and spicy English mustard should be combined in a separate bowl. Squeeze some mayonnaise and mustard on top of the cooked chicken. Butter the bread with the unsalted butter. Grill the sandwich by placing the chicken on one slice of bread, then putting the second slice on top.

Seafood Salad with Prawn, Crab, and Lobster - 429 Calorie Choice

Cleaning and barbecuing six King Prawns.

Four tablespoons of fresh, cooked crab flesh per serving

Freshly cooked lobster flesh, approximately 4 tablespoons.

3 capers, minced

1 tsp of jalapeño peppers

2 tbsp. olives, chopped

14 cups mixed salad greens, chopped

2 tablespoons of feta cheese

a quarter of an avocado, diced

> 1 tbsp. toasted sesame seeds

3 tablespoons of low-fat mayo

A half-cup of Dijon mustard, grated

1 tbsp of organic balsamic vinegar

1 tsp of tomato ketchup /

Organic honey, 1 tbsp.

Combine the low-fat mayo, Dijon mustard, ketchup, honey, and balsamic vinegar in a small mixing basin. Toss the salad ingredients, including the fish, in a large bowl. Enjoy the mustard salad dressing drizzled over the salad.

Grilled Portobello Mushrooms with Feta Cheese and an Avocado Bun -

Calories in 500

1 big portobello mushroom /

(about 1 tablespoon)

As much as you'd want!

At least a pound of chips

2 tbsp. olives, chopped

Salt and pepper to taste (low sodium)

Make sure the stalk side is facing up on a cooking pan before placing it on the grill. Toss the mushrooms with garlic flakes, a pinch of sea salt, and feta cheese crumbles. Place it on the grill and heat it until it begins to soften and the feta has melted, then remove it. Using a knife, remove the avocado's skin and split it in half lengthwise. Remove the tip from the mushroom and set it on the avocado half that has been cut in half. Using the other half of the avocado, make an avocado burger by covering the mushroom with the avocado. 1 cup of tortilla chips and as much spiciness as required can be served as a starter.

Chapter Four

My personal recipes

Ideas for a Healthy Dinner

It's important to eat well during dinner, especially if you plan to fast the next day or all night into the next day. Avoid going to bed with a full stomach by eating earlier in the evening. A full stomach is difficult to digest and can cause sleep issues.

Non-Limited Calorie Fasting

This might be your second meal of the day during a fasting phase, depending on your eating window. Non-fasting healthy meal ideas may be found under the non-fasting healthy ideas section. Once again, use self-control and gradually reduce your serving portions. It's better to eat more during lunch than at evening.

It's best to avoid eating after 7:30 pm every night.

calorie-restricted fasting (170 to 250 Calories)

The following are some of the best low-calorie supper options on the market, all of which are delicious and nutritious.

Chickpea Burger with Ham and Cottage Cheese - 250 Calories

2 buns of whole wheat patty

2 tbsp fat-free cottage cheese and 1 tbsp minced cooked ham

1/4 cup chickpeas mashed

54   THE BENEFITS OF KETO AND INTERMITTENT DIET FOR 50+

2 heads of lettuce

14 tsp of a spicy pepper sauce

Drain the chickpeas, then mash them with a potato masher. Serve with more spicy sauce and ham on the side for a complete meal. Form the chickpea mixture into a patty by patting it out into a round shape. Chickpea patties can be grilled for 8 to 10 minutes, or until they're cooked through. Slice the burger bread in half and top each half with a lettuce leaf. Put the chickpea patties on the bottom half of the burger, then seal the two parts together and eat it up!

239 Calorie Recipe: One Potato Mash with Grilled Tuna

1 boiling and mashed Idaho potato

1 piece of grilled tuna

1 cup of baby spinach

One tablespoon of pine nuts.

feta cheese, 1 tablespoon

One teaspoon of sunflower seeds

1 tbsp. cashew nuts, chopped raw

2 tbsp of organic balsamic vinegar /

Toss the tuna on the grill with black pepper and low-sodium salt. The Idaho potato may be boiled and mashed. Then sprinkle balsamic vinegar over the greens and top with the feta cheese and pine nuts. The tuna should be served on top of the mash, with the green salad on the side.

A serving of the Vegetable and 3 Cheese Tart has 215 calories.

12 of an eggplant

three courgettes

Approximately a 12-ounce can of sweet cherry tomatoes

> 12 cup young spinach leaves

Two tablespoons of chopped olive slices

MY PERSONAL RECIPES 55

One tablespoon of chopped jalapeño peppers

Puff pastry, one (1) roll

A quarter cup of feta

• 4 tbsp fat-free yoghurt

2 tbsp of parmesan This is plent for three people.

Set the oven temperature to 300°F. A baking pan should be coated in cooking spray. A pie crust made of filo pastry should be laid out in an even layer on the baking sheet. In a preheated oven, bake the pastry until golden brown. Over medium heat, sauté the veggies in a pan with coconut oil. Once the meat and vegetables have been cooked, add the cream cheese and put them in the pie shell. Sprinkle feta cheese on top of the vegetables and olives. Bake for a further 8 to 10 minutes, or until the cheese has melted, then top with a sprinkle of parmesan. Serve immediately after taking it out of the oven.

218 Calories - Asparagus, Green Bean, and Poached Egg Salad

5 spears of fresh grilled asparagus

Grilled green beans, approximately 1 cup in volume

2 eggs poached in a pan

> 12 cup young spinach leaves

a quarter cup of rocket

3-4 tablespoons of Dijon mustard

Lay a mixture of baby spinach and rocket leaves on a flat surface. Stack the mixed leaves with the grilled asparagus and beans. Poach an egg and then sprinkle with Dijon mustard on top of the salad.

Boiled Garlic and Ginger Butter Baby grilled turkey breast

There are 250 calories in a serving of potatoes.

4 tiny potatoes, cleaned and cooked

Cut one turkey breast in half and serve it in slices.

1 tbsp freshly grated ginger

2 cloves organic smashed garlic, minced finely.

3 tbsp of unsalted butter.

black pepper and low-sodium salt to taste

Serve the cooked baby potatoes beside the grilled and sliced turkey breast. In a small saucepan, combine the butter, ginger, and garlic, and heat through. To eat, simply drizzle the butter mixture on top of the tiny potatoes and enjoy. If you like, you can toss in some mixed salad greens.

Normal Eating Day Dinner Ideas (500 Calories and Under)

These recipes are quick and easy to prepare, contain less than 500 calories, and are packed with nutrients.

a Cajun Baked Potato Wedges with Sour Cream Bison Burger

- 500 kcal per serving

At least one patties of bison.

1 whole-wheat hamburger bun

1 Tbsp Mustard with a hint of Dijon flavour

1 big pickle, cut into thin strips

A single big, thoroughly cleaned lettuce leaf

1 medium-sized tomato

1 cup cooked potato wedges, sliced thinly

1 tsp Cajun seasoning.

Sour cream: 3 Tbsp Low Fat

1 tbsp. fresh dill, chopped finely

Spread Dijon mustard on both halves of the burger bun before slicing in half. It is best to grill your bison burger before you stack it on the bottom half of the bun.

MY PERSONAL RECIPES   57

bun. Add a lettuce leaf, a tomato slice, and a sliced pickle to the burger before serving. Sour cream and dill should be combined in a bowl. Add Cajun spice to the sour cream and chive sauce before baking the potato wedges as instructed.

Baked Potato and Sour Cream with Seafood and Turf - 500 Calories

1 thick-cut prime steak, grilled and seasoned to taste

cooked to tenderness for one big baking potato

6 grilled prawns in a big pot

garlic butter, 1 tblsp

One teaspoon of unsalted butter

Sour cream, 1 tablespoon

1 cup of boiled green beans.

Serve with your favourite steak sauce and baked potato. When the prawns are almost done cooking, heat the butter and garlic in a skillet. The green beans should be cooked to your preference and then placed on a dinner dish. You may also serve it with baked potatoes and seared steak. Pour the prawns with the warm garlic butter on top. Add sour cream, salt, and pepper to the baked potato and serve it while it's still warm.

An easy black bean chilli with only 343 calories per serving

14 cup of brown rice that has been cooked

A quarter of a white onion finely sliced

2 medium-sized fresh tomatoes

1 can of black beans / black beans

garlic, crushed, 2 tbsp.

chile powder, about 1 tbsp (strength to your taste)

2 tbsp of honey made from organic sources.

jalapeño jalapenos, about two tablespoons

The vinegar should be organic and of high quality. 2 tablespoons

2 tsp of paprika

2 tbsp. sour cream

4 tbsp feta cheese

avocado, thinly sliced: 12

8 fresh mint sprigs

Warm water, 14 cup

There are four servings in this recipe.

Cook the rice fifteen minutes before the chilli is done cooking. Add the onion, black beans, smashed garlic, chilli powder, honey, balsamic vinegar, and paprika to the boiling water in a big saucepan. 1 hour 30 minutes, or until the beans are mushy enough. If you want to go all out, garnish with some fresh mint and feta crumbled on top of your guacamole.

Pizza with avocado, bacon, kale, and feta is 342 calories.

The equivalent of one whole wheat tortilla would be

14 avocado sliced thinly

14 cup of drained and crisped bacon

> 4 tablespoons rocket

A little amount of feta cheese (around 2 tablespoons)

2 cups shredded parmesan

Tomato paste made with organic ingredients, 2 tablespoons

black pepper and low-sodium salt to taste

Set the oven temperature to 340°F. On top of the tortilla, spread the tomato paste and top it with feta cheese. Cook in the oven until the tortilla is golden brown and the filling is hot.

Pancakes with Spicy Mince Meat - 370 Calories

MY PERSONAL RECIPES 59

Preparation: 2 eggs, 14 cup flour, 14 cup fat-free milk for pancakes

The equivalent of one cup of minced meat

5 basil fronds

Dried oregano, 1 teaspoon

Chilli powder can be substituted with the ground pepper.

One tablespoon of jalapeño peppers

At least a tablespoon of capers

14 cup of mixed salad greens

14 cucumber, finely diced

1 sliced celery stalk

One tablespoon of balsamic vinegar

You should make a pair of pancakes. Gather your spices and herbs and add them to the mince. Dish the mince out equally into the centre of each pancake. Add jalapeño peppers and capers to each pancake and serve. Then, apply balsamic vinegar over the salad greens (cucumber, celery, and salad leaves).

As a side dish, serve the pancakes with a green salad.

Smoothies that are nutritious

Breakfast or lunch may be swapped out for one of these delicious smoothies. In addition, they can be eaten as a snack.

Fruit, nut, and vegetable combinations abound in the world of smoothie making. Add a variety of nut milks, creams, yoghurts, and so on to your smoothie recipe. When you add seeds, they become infinitely more delectable.

The components should be nutritious and within the recommended snack or meal calorie intake. They're a terrific method to make sure you're getting in all of your daily dietary needs. They may be eaten as a quick supper or snack while on the run.

If you want to drink a smoothie, you must do it at mealtimes or during designated drinking windows. They cannot be consumed during fasting times since they are a snack that contains carbohydrates.

Put all of the ingredients into a blender and mix until smooth and thick, and you've got a delicious smoothie. Smoothie leftovers keep well in the refrigerator for up to two days if stored in an airtight container.

Protein powder may be added to smoothies to help with muscle recovery after a workout, such as a long run, a bike ride, etc. If you're feeling drained and rundown, they might offer you an extra surge of energy.

During Fasting Periods, Beverages

When fasting, some beverages can be consumed, while others must be avoided. During a fast, certain ingredients must be avoided, while others can be included.

The following are some suggestions on what you should and should not drink during fasting.

Water

Even if you are not fasting, you should drink water throughout the day.

Natural, filtered, or spring water that can be either carbonated or still is always the finest option for drinking water.

You are welcome to add your own.

▯ Lemon

▯ Lime

Slices of cucumber.

Carbonation is an option for the water.

You are not allowed to submit any other information.

Sweeteners synthesised in a lab

▯ Colorants

Flavors synthesised in a lab

MY PERSONAL RECIPES

☐ Fruit

☐ Berries

Tea

A few teas should be avoided, while others are OK to drink. If the tea has to be cooled down, it's best to drink it black with a splash of ice water.

Alternatively, you might sip on one of the following beverages.

Tea oolong

Tea in the form of black tea

Tea that isn't flavoured.

Tea, specifically, green tea.

Cinnamon flavoured tea

A cup of tea with peppermint

A cup of tea brewed with spearmint

You are welcome to add your own.

☐ Stevia

☐ Cinnamon

☐ Nutmeg

Juice of one lemon

You are not allowed to submit any other information.

Sweeteners synthesised in a lab

☐ Milk

☐ Cream

Flavors synthesised in a lab

☐ Fruit

- Herbs

- Spices

Coffee

You can stay awake and attentive by drinking a cup of black coffee. It can also help you lose weight.

You are welcome to add your own.

- Stevia

- Cinnamon

- Nutmeg

Juice of one lemon

You are not allowed to submit any other information.

Sweeteners synthesised in a lab

- Milk

- Cream

Flavors synthesised in a lab

- Herbs

- Spices

Fasting-Related Anxieties

They suffer migraines, feel sick, or are unable to keep their hunger at bay when fasting. The following advice will help alleviate some of your fears.

Constipation

Fasting can cause constipation, especially when you're just getting started.

Here are some ideas to get you started:

During the times when you're most likely to eat, try to up your fibre intake.

MY PERSONAL RECIPES 63

Consume carbonated water.

The seeds can be added to smoothies or sprinkled on meals.

Have a cup of hot coffee.

Black or green tea are good options.

Dizziness

During the fasting periods, you may experience dizziness or vertigo. A blood rush to the head or standing up may also cause you to feel dizzy. When this happens, it's typically because you've been drinking too little water.

Here are some ideas to get you started:

Drink more fluids to stay hydrated.

Mint can be added to your water at the mealtimes.

Eat only when you have a window of opportunity to take liver salts.

For a period, stop drinking coffee and tea.

Lethargy or exhaustion

Fatigue and lethargy are common side effects of fasting. Perhaps your body isn't getting enough of the nutrients it needs. When you're not fasting, up your nutritional intake.

Here are some ideas to get you started:

Drink more fluids to stay hydrated.

At least an hour before your fasting period is due to begin, consume high-energy items during your window of eating.

Spray your face with some icy water.

Do some modest physical activity.

Take your vitamins when you are eating.

Headaches

During fasting, headaches are a regular occurrence. Because it is not used to being deprived of food, your body will experience withdrawal symptoms.

Here are some ideas to get you started:

Increase your water intake.

During your non-fasting intervals, drink mineral water.

Anxiety-induced muscle twitches or twitches

Cutting out on salt and other minerals is also part of fasting. Muscle spasms and cramps are possible side effects.

Here are some ideas to get you started:

Make sure you take Epsom salts twice a week throughout your meal times.

Make sure you're getting enough magnesium during your mealtimes.

Nausea

Feeling hungry can cause nausea, and migraines can cause nausea as well.

Here are some ideas to get you started:

Take a cup of peppermint tea.

During the time when you should be eating, consume liver salts.

Hunger

Feeling hungry is the most prevalent source of anxiety or dissatisfaction. There is a lot you can do to alleviate your hunger sensations and prevent you from feeling hungry in the first place.

Here are some ideas to get you started:

During the times when you're most likely to eat, try to up your fibre intake.

At least an hour before the fasting phase begins, eat extra slow-releasing carbohydrates.

Consume carbonated water.

Drinking green tea is recommended.

MY PERSONAL RECIPES 65

Have a cup of joe.

Cinnamon may be added to coffee or tea to enhance the flavour.

Keep yourself occupied with a pastime.

Take a short stroll or do some mild exercise.

☑ Meditate.

Visit a close buddy.

Affecting Your Sleep

If you're fasting through the night, you've probably been fasting since 7:30 p.m. or so, at the latest. Having a small snack and a cup of chamomile tea before going to bed is recommended.

Turn off any technological devices that might disrupt your sleep cycle while you read a book. Make sure your room is cold, especially in the winter, so that you can get a good night's sleep.

Keep a bottle of water next to your bed so that you don't have to get up and go pour one yourself if you become thirsty at night.

Learn sleep meditation techniques to help you fall asleep more easily and get a good night's rest.

Getting What You Want

Remember that what you put into your body has a direct impact on how you feel, as the old adage goes. While on the Keto diet, your body is accumulating energy reserves that it may use whenever it needs them. As a result, you should notice an increase in your energy and stamina, allowing you to get through each day with ease. No more sluggishness, which is a common side effect of other diets. When you're on Keto, you're supposed to have more energy and a limitless amount of potential. In the long run, your diet will no longer seem like a diet at all. In time, you will discover that eating a Keto diet is truly enjoyable. Your body's metabolism will change, which will lead to a change in what it desires. Keep in mind that your body will ultimately need fat and protein as you proceed on the Keto diet.

It's important to keep track of your progress.

It is usually a good idea to compare and contrast one's development. Take a moment to reflect on how you felt before beginning the Keto diet. Now would be a good moment to start a journal, if you haven't already. Keep a journal where you may jot down your moods and desires. It's also possible to record your weight and BMI. You'll be able to utilise this data as a source of inspiration if you have concrete numbers to work with. As you complete another day of the Keto diet, allow yourself to feel a sense of accomplishment. Commit to the diet and to yourself. This will provide its own set of difficulties, but you won't be thrown off course by them.

Have faith in your capacity to see this through.

You are what you eat.

Take a step back and remember what it was like to satisfy your sweet and calorie-laden desires. However, it's important to keep in mind the wider picture when answering this question. Is it true that these foods made you feel more energised? Did you feel a lull in energy after eating them? Getting what you want right away may seem good at the time, but you'll likely have to live with the repercussions afterwards. It's merely a temporary fix to satisfy your desires if you eat junk food. Reinforcing the habit also trains your body to crave these substances. You won't burn calories or utilise sugar as a source of energy if you eat junk food, which has little nutritious value. Think about it, you really don't need this junk stuff.

Recognize that there are alternatives to relying on food to make you happy. Eating with others might be a lot of fun, but it's not the only thing about food that makes you happy. When you are certain that you are taking care of your body, you may choose to be joyful. Enjoy the feeling of knowing that you're providing your body with food it can genuinely use. Keto-friendly cuisine may not provide the same instant high as junk food, but the long-term benefits far outweigh the short-term ones. What matters most is that you will be able to see its effects long after you've eaten the food. In order to recognise that your happiness isn't related to the things you eat, all you need is a simple shift in your perspective. Your contentment must come from a more profound source.

It's common for people to turn to food for consolation when they're feeling unhappy or anxious. Many people view this as a cultural norm. You will learn how to deal with your emotions in a way that isn't dependent on the foods you eat while on the Keto diet. When you've had a tough day, the Keto diet teaches you to fuel yourself instead of giving in to your cravings. A healthy diet might help you feel more energised and keep your endorphins in check. You already know that this will be enough to lift your spirits whenever you feel down. It's a long-term answer for those issues that seem to resurface again and again. It's much simpler to remember why you're on the Keto diet if you approach it from this angle.

No diet should cause you to feel so terrible that you can't even appreciate the benefits of your new lifestyle.. in no way should following a ketogenic diet make you feel as if you have no other alternatives. While on the Keto diet, you should really experience the reverse. With so little to lose, you should be able to prepare a wide variety of meals that you may enjoy without feeling guilty. Even if you're eating a nutritious diet, you should avoid diets that cause you mental distress. Mental well-being is equally as critical as physical health. Your degree of contentment will plummet if your state of mind begins to degrade. When you're on a diet, you're permitted to be joyful. The first sign that things isn't right is when you begin to feel depressed.

More and more people will understand that Keto doesn't have to be restrictive or tough because of your example. Keeping the diet grounded in reality might be as simple as being able to explain it to others. The fact that you're able to keep to a diet while also seeming cheerful and content will serve as an example to your loved ones. You may have tried to imitate this feeling in the past when on a diet, but the Keto diet does not need any such trickery. Identifying exactly what is making you feel the way you do is essential. In the event you begin to feel unwell, it is recommended you change your diet until you feel better. The Keto diet is supposed to be easy on the body.

Things Will Get Better for You

At some point on the Keto diet, you go from attempting to succeeding to really succeeding. You're certain to experience this at some time in your life, so savour the moment. Focusing on the fact that you're following a diet isn't always a bad thing; instead, it's a good thing. Make sure you're having fun with your life! As there are so many things in this world that aim to drag you down, it's important to focus on the things that truly lift you up. It's one of the first benefits of the Keto diet that will help you feel more energised. It's expected that you'll begin to see this benefit as soon as you get started. Invest your energy in the most efficient manner possible. Keeping in mind that the diet has given you a little extra fuel for the day, split your time carefully.

Try to maintain healthy habits, such as going to bed and waking up early, even if your energy levels appear to be increasing. This is going to help you better control your internal processes. Keeping in mind that the Keto diet will offer you a boost of energy is the key to success. It's your responsibility to stay on top of things. It's almost as though these advantages are being thrown away if you do nothing with them. In order to reap the benefits, you must be aware of them at all times. When you first start recognising these new changes, make an effort to practise as many good behaviours as you can. You're in for an exciting and energising period right now!

You'll Become a New Person.

You'll notice a difference in your look as one of the next advantages you'll begin to experience. Your skin should have a young radiance and a healthy shine about it. Feeling embarrassed about your skin as you get older can have a significant negative influence on your self-esteem. Don't worry about it, since your body is doing exactly what it was designed to accomplish. There is no way to avoid ageing, but the Keto diet can make the process easier. When you begin to see improvements in the appearance of your skin, it is time to commit to better skin care practises. Always wash your face before going to bed, use sunscreen, and moisturise regularly. Having a good skincare regimen doesn't need a lot of time or money, so do your best to care for your skin.

Keto's weight loss potential is one of the most eagerly awaited aspects of the diet. First, you'll feel a rush of exhilaration flood over you. Losing weight and staying healthy will become a personal battle. This weight reduction isn't simply a one-time occurrence because you'll be consuming genuine fat. Keeping the weight off will be a breeze as long as you stick to the Keto diet. Many other diets promise rapid weight reduction, but this is just a result of water loss or, even worse, muscle loss. A disappointing effect might be the fact that this excess weight is so much simpler to regain.

Regardless of why you started the Keto diet, your body will start to thin down as a result of it. Time your workouts correctly and make sure you're receiving enough exercise each week if you want to grow muscle. Your training will be more enjoyable if you know what kind of exercise you prefer. You shouldn't have to do a bodybuilder's exercise if you're not a bodybuilder. It wouldn't be logical. It's important to make sure that your training routine is tailored to your current lifestyle and skill level. In the future, if you desire, you may always tweak it to make it more difficult.

Keto is a great way to improve your culinary skills, which is something many people fail to realise when they first begin the diet. Preparing everything yourself is much more convenient because your meals will need to be adjusted. Aside from occasional take-out, you'll discover that cooking may be a reward-

MY PERSONAL RECIPES   69

ing experience. You'll discover new methods to prepare familiar dishes as well as new ways to flavour them. Even if you've never cooked before, you should be able to put up a basic Keto meal plan that doesn't need a lot of effort. If you put in the time and effort, you may even be able to cook the same meals for other members of your family.

You are not who you are as a person because of what you eat. As a result, while on Keto, you may still take pleasure in all aspects of your life. Eating habits account for a significant element of one's psyche, yet they are not the sum whole of one's existence. Consider all of your positive attributes outside of your Keto eating habits. When you respect yourself more, you'll be able to recognise that Keto is just going to bring you more benefits. Even if you don't follow this diet, there are many wonderful things about you to be proud of. When you're trying to stick to your diet, it's best to keep these two items distinct to avoid feelings of guilt or failure. You should be aware that there is no diet worth sacrificing your self-esteem for.

You'll be able to become the most successful version of yourself if you have a positive connection with diets. You won't get the greatest benefits if you start the Keto diet and hate it. Eating well shouldn't be a source of worry in your life; instead, it should be a source of joy. When it comes to dieting, many people are taught that they must fight their diet to succeed. Keto is unique in that it eliminates the need for such an uphill battle. As long as you pay attention to what your body and mind are telling you, you should only experience good feelings.

If you're still not sure if the Keto diet is right for you, keep in mind everything we've covered thus far to help you decide. Does your life still allow you to experience these benefits in the way you prefer? Whenever you find yourself feeling constrained, it is because you are imposing your own self-imposed limitations on yourself. Keep a positive attitude if you see yourself getting down in the dumps. When you follow the Keto diet, you'll be able to demonstrate to yourself that it's doable without adhering to a rigid set of rules. Remind yourself that you are a complete person, regardless of whether you are on a diet or not. You shouldn't let going keto define who you are; instead, let it highlight all of your best traits. You'll be able to tell that you're prospering once you comprehend this. Sensation good about yourself when you're achieving your goals is a wonderful feeling.

It's important that your work inspires others, but it should also inspire you. Reward yourself for making it to your goal and acknowledge the difficulties you had along the way. Being on a diet might be difficult at first, but you'll quickly adjust to the Keto diet. You'll wonder what you ever ate before you started this diet. That's why most people stick with Keto for good. Even those who agree to give it a try for a few months do so for a significantly longer period of time. If it's still working for you, don't stop. With all of the health advantages you've come to expect in addition to the joy of eating clean foods, you're more than likely to continue to feel fantastic while on Keto.

Optimism fills you

The Keto diet can help you become acclimated to having a more positive outlook on life. Positivity permeates all part of one's life when one practises it. You will always meet obstacles and disappointments in your life, but keeping a positive attitude can help you overcome them. When you're older, it's more difficult to make amends for mistakes, which can be frustrating. Being healthy and reducing weight can be two of those things. It will be difficult to have a positive outlook if you no longer believe that you can achieve specific goals. Here are some of the benefits of the Keto diet for you. Everything it does for your body corresponds with a positive attitude.

Pessimism has no place in your life now that you're putting your health and well-being first.

It's a good idea to examine your life before starting a diet. Think about how you deal with unpleasant situations in your life. When you discover that your coping mechanisms are based on eating badly or not obtaining adequate nutrients, you may understand that your coping skills are lacking. Don't blame yourself for these tendencies; instead, look for them. You'll have a better sense of what needs to be changed once you've identified them. It is easier to make positive changes in your life if you are able to look at yourself objectively and with an open mind. Admit that you may not have the best coping skills right now, but that you can improve your situation if you want to.

Think about what you actually desire for yourself and for your life. Take a step back and think about things that don't provide you immediate pleasure. It's critical that you take your time with this, since it may be a profound epiphany. To keep your thoughts in order, you may either meditate or write them down. Try to focus solely on the things that will help you achieve your objectives. You'll be able to focus on what's most essential by letting go of the belief that quick solutions would assist you. It's tough to get to the bottom of these things, but knowing where you are in your life right now is helpful. As you embark on your Keto adventure, all of this matters.

MY PERSONAL RECIPES 71

Commit yourself to changing your unhealthy behaviours and establishing new ones in their stead. There is less sense of giving up when there is a solution in sight. Instead, it's like you're simply changing the way you think. In order to maintain a positive outlook while on the Ketogenic diet, you should follow these tips. Never deprive yourself of food or anything else without first considering a worthwhile substitute. As a result of this method, you will never feel like you are missing out on the things in your life that you truly desire. Instead, you'll be educating your mind and body to crave better foods.

Happiness and food are more intertwined than you would imagine! In addition to consuming meals that make you feel better when you are down, there are some foods that are healthy for your brain and so naturally increase your level of pleasure. You can keep your brain active and bright by eating these meals, which are usually high in protein. Like any other muscle in your body, your brain grows weak and fatigued if it is not regularly exercised. As a result, doing so becomes a bother because it no longer works as well as it did in the past. Regular consumption of omega-3-rich proteins and healthy fats will provide your brain with the energy it needs to function properly. It will be in peak physical condition and performing at its best. You'll be happy because you'll know exactly what you're doing and how you're feeling.

Having a clouded mind might make life more difficult. The cloud of doubt that looms over you might cause you to believe that something is amiss, even if it isn't. If you're not careful, your brain might lead you to a lot of different conclusions. If you're starting to feel depressed, you should take a close look at your food. It may seem insignificant, yet it has a significant impact on how your brain functions. Even though you're dealing with personal difficulties, they aren't your sole difficulty. Eating junk food and preservatives deprives your body of the necessary nutrients for the production of happy brain chemicals. You'll have to feed it til you crash, then restart the process on sugar.

Having a rudimentary understanding of how the brain works is essential if you want to stay positive while following the Keto diet. If you aren't consuming foods that are rich in nutrients, it will be more difficult to keep a happy brain. Make note of how your head feels and how clear your ideas are after your first week on protein. You'll probably notice that your thoughts are lot more focused and you have a greater sense of self-assurance. Giving your brain the opportunity to function as it was designed to does wonders for mental health and well-being. This is critical for everyone, as a life without direction can lead to feelings of hopelessness and sadness. It's not uncommon for people to have feelings of helplessness and terror as a result of this. When you're on Keto, you have an automatic reason to get out of bed every morning. As soon as you begin to see the favourable effects of the diet on your cognitive function, this is just one more reason to include it into your daily routine.

Keeping a Positive Attitude

Everything you accomplish in life should be fueled by a sense of purpose and wonder. You'll be more driven to achieve your objectives if you have someone to look up to for inspiration. To begin your adventure on the Keto diet, this guide might serve as an inspiration. You should be pumped up and eager to get started now that you've learned about the lifestyle's many advantages. When you get the hang of the Keto diet, you begin to inspire yourself. Maintaining a regular schedule can help you achieve this goal.

Routines are a part of everyone's daily life, whether they're constantly shifting or staying the same. Routines provide you a sense of security and predictability, both of which are beneficial! In order to stay on track, you need a regimen that is both regular and adaptable. The best routines provide for plenty of space for error and, if required, modification.

Recite positive affirmations to yourself each morning as you begin your day. As basic as "I can accomplish this" or as elaborate as you choose, these affirmations are all up to you. No matter what is going on in your life, you can always return to optimism if you start the day with a positive outlook. Use your morning meal as an opportunity to appreciate the fact that you're feeding your body. There is no better way to start the day than with a healthy Keto breakfast. Make sure your lunch is packed and ready to go if you are taking it to work. As a result, you will no longer have to worry about what to have for lunch on that day. The better your day goes, the more stresses you can minimise.

As soon as lunch is served, take the time to enjoy every mouthful. Take a seat and savour your meal. Be inspired by the quality and therapeutic powers of the food that you consume. You should just utilise your lunch break to eat and nothing else. Your body won't be able to rest if you're doing many things at once. As you eat your lunch, all of the strain and stress that you've been carrying about all morning will be with you. You may have bloating, gas, or indigestion as a result of your digestive system acting up. When you're under a lot of pressure, tension builds up in your stomach, which has the potential to affect your eating habits. Don't worry about what's going on in the outside world. You'll be allowed to go back after lunch. What a difference a few moments of calm can make to your day after you've been dealing with a lot of stress all day.

MY PERSONAL RECIPES 73

If you do get the chance to go out to eat with your friends while on the Keto diet, make it a point to prove to them that you know what you're doing. Is there any way to make typical restaurant cuisine healthier? It's okay to be concerned about your health, and you shouldn't feel bad about it. On a diet, you may still have fun and be happy despite the restrictions. It's designed to become a part of your daily routine. Friends and family members should be sympathetic to your plight and willing to lend a helping hand. The people who care about you the most will not be able to make you feel guilty about following the Keto diet if you show them how amazing it makes you feel. Make sure you know who you're spending time with at this difficult time. For a successful trip, you need a supportive group of people who can inspire and encourage your progress. Your friends and family may even begin to consider the diet as something they would like to try for themselves.

By now, you've probably been able to get past some of the negative connotations associated with following a Ketogenic diet. For the last few decades, dieting has been a contentious issue in society, and this is true of any diet plan. Doing everything you can to educate others about the benefits of the keto diet is the most important thing you can do. Changing people's minds about how the Keto diet works may be accomplished by showing them that they aren't actually "starving" and that they are reaping the advantages of weight reduction and increased energy. As long as you stick to what you know, you'll be able to keep experiencing the positive outcomes you're looking for. People are naturally dubious.

Take advantage of the opportunity to try something new during dinner time. Dinner should be different every night, whether you're dining at home or going out to a new restaurant, so that you don't become bored.

Given the elements that Keto promotes, there are a plethora of possibilities for what you can produce. All of your meals will be filled with protein and taste. Cooking with butter and oil allows you to recreate all of your favourite meals without having to exclude any ingredients. The Keto diet's rules contain many of the foods that people like most. It's almost too wonderful to be true, say some individuals, that they can still consume these foods! Inspiration comes from eating meals that are good for you.

Doing something for your health, such as exercising, may be a source of inspiration for you and your actions. On a new diet, getting up and exercising might be a challenge. Congratulations on your hard work at the gym. The Keto diet will have you seeing results in no time, so keep it up. You'll be more inclined to

74 THE BENEFITS OF KETO AND INTERMITTENT DIET FOR 50+

return to these behaviours in the future if you get into them now. In time, they become less of a chore and more of a part of your daily routine. Keto should seem simple and natural once you get into the swing of things.

Conclusion

Now that you've learned so much about the Keto diet, you should be ready to embark on your own Keto adventure with confidence. Keeping this in mind as you begin to change your lifestyle and alter your eating habits can help you stay on track with your weight loss goals. Your body will undergo a shift as it learns to use the excellent fats and protein in this diet as energy. You'll be able to tap into your body's reservoir of energy whenever you need it. It's already inside of you, whether you need it for a morning pick-me-up or a boost to get you through the day.

With your anti-aging goals in mind, you may enjoy the benefits of the Keto diet while you take care of yourself over the next several years. It not only keeps you looking and feeling younger, but it also serves as a protective barrier against a variety of illnesses and disorders.. By providing you with a constant supply of energy-burning and muscle-building chances, Keto helps to protect your body against deterioration. When it comes to Keto, you just take what you have an abundance of, rather than what you need to feel wonderful. This is how you'll always feel your best on a daily basis, no matter what.

Keto is one of the finest diets out there since you have so many alternatives for meals! You may eat a wide variety of tasty and full meals on any of the Keto diet regimens. Even if you go out to eat, you can still stick to this diet by bringing it along. Remembering the fundamental rules of Keto is all that's required to keep your diet on track. As your body strives to alter the way it digests, cravings disappear nearly completely. Your body shifts its attention from depending on glucose in the bloodstream. As soon as you achieve ketosis, your body begins to burn fat. The greatest part is, you do not have to do anything other than eating within your fat/protein/carb ratios. Your body will accomplish the rest on its own.

Keto is more than just a trendy diet since it allows your body to function effectively for lengthy periods of time. Originating with a medical basis for assisting epilepsy sufferers, the Keto diet has been researched and tested for decades. Research shows that Keto works, and it's supported by a number of research. Dieting for a month or a year is just as beneficial for your health. Keto is a lifestyle change, but it's one you'll reap the rewards of for as long as you're willing to stick with it. Because of this, if you're ready to feel and look your best from head to toe, you can begin your Keto journey with confidence. Keto dieters may overcome the natural ageing process and hormonal abnormalities that come with being a woman by adhering to the diet in a balanced way. Change your life and reap the advantages of a Keto diet now.

CPSIA information can be obtained
at www.ICGtesting.com
Printed in the USA
LVHW062310030822
724960LV00010BB/514